# Reflective Practice in Nursing

6E

# Reflective Practice in Nursing

6E

Annemarie Horn

LM

Learning Matters
A Sage Publishing Company

3rd Floor, HYLO
103-105 Bunhill Row
London, EC1Y 8LZ

2455 Teller Road
Thousand Oaks
California 91320

10th Floor, Emaar Capital Tower 2
MG Road, Sikanderpur, Sector 26
Gurugram, Haryana – 122002
India

8 Marina View Suite 43-053
Asia Square Tower 1
Singapore 018960

Editor: Laura Walmsley
Editorial Assistant: Sahar Jamfar
Senior project editor: Chris Marke
Project manager: TNQ Tech Pvt. Ltd.
Marketing manager: Ruslana Khatagova
Cover design: Sheila Tong
Typeset by: TNQ Tech Pvt. Ltd.
Printed in the UK



**A Library of Congress Control Number is available for this title.**

**British Library Cataloguing in Publication Data**

A catalogue record for this book is available from the British Library

ISBN 978-1-0362-0932-2
ISBN 978-1-0362-0931-5 (pbk)

# Contents

# Foreword

The Transforming Nursing Practice series includes several titles that focus on developing nurses' personal and professional learning skills. Reflective Practice in Nursing is a great example in this respect. Life-long learning in nursing involves a constant dialogue between nurses' personal inner world and the outer scientific, technological and cultural world of professional practice. This book carefully and skilfully shows the reader how to incorporate all of these different strands within their professional identity and development as nurses through reflective practice. High-quality care links personal attributes such as self-awareness with professional expertise in delivering reflective, empathetic, person-centred and evidence-based nursing care. Each chapter is loaded with interesting case studies and learning activities to engage readers in reflection whilst developing their self-awareness, problem-solving skills and nursing knowledge that is grounded in the realities of clinical practice. After reading this book, both nursing students and registered nurses will be well informed in applying the principles of reflective practice to review and learn from their interactions with patients. It will also enhance their personal and professional development in addressing key Nursing and Midwifery Council (NMC) standards to deliver safe, effective and compassionate care.

The sixth edition has been updated to reflect developments in nursing and healthcare, sources of knowledge and references and feedback received from readers and reviewers. A modified reflective framework is also presented to help demystify the process. The changes refresh the book's focus on collaborative, sensitive, inclusive, thoughtful, adaptive, relevant, effective and person-centred reflective nursing practice that respects individual and cultural differences. Hence, Reflective Practice in Nursing remains an essential guide in the professional development of nurses to enhance better patient care through reflective practice.

*Dr Mooi Standing*
*Series Editor*

# Acknowledgements

This work reflects four decades of nursing experience, clinically and academically. I dedicate the book to everyone I have ever met on this journey, specifically those who allowed me to grow, reflect and broaden my reflective knowledge and understanding.

Professional thanks to Caroline Yorke and Angela Jackson for sharing their emotional intelligence and compassion in every reflective discussion. Thanks to my mother Patty for teaching me how to see many sides of an experience from an early age and to Bruce Horn for continuing on with this gift in our life together.

Thanks also to Dr Mooi Standing for her helpful suggestions in the editing of the chapters. I would also like to thank my editors at Sage.

# Publisher's acknowledgements

We would like to acknowledge the hard work of Dr Lioba Howatson-Jones in first conceiving and writing this text for Learning Matters. We would also like to acknowledge and thank Dr Philip Esterhuizen for updating the book in its fourth and fifth editions. Over the course of various editions, this work has helped many students to understand the importance of reflection in their practice and to develop their reflective skills, and we are grateful that this text can continue to help students for many editions to come.

# About the authors

**Annemarie Horn** was a Senior Lecturer in the Institute of Health at the University of Cumbria where she taught undergraduate and postgraduate students. Working with a strong moral compass, she encouraged reflective practice and ethical awareness to help the individual student to develop their caring attitudes.

With professional experience in the Northwest of England, Guernsey and Alderney, her work included remote healthcare, where dementia became her focus; as she wished to understand individual experiences to enable the provision of safe, kind, and effective care in the support of patients and families.

This sixth edition has been updated by Annemarie from the original work by Lioba Howatson-Jones.

**Dr Lioba Howatson-Jones** was a Senior Lecturer in the School of Nursing at Canterbury Christ Church University, where she taught pre-registration, post-registration, master's and PhD students. Lioba's clinical nursing background is mainly in acute and radiology nursing and practice development. Her research interests are in exploring nurses' learning and academic development. Lioba has published on these and clinical topics since 1999.

# Introduction

This book provides suggestions for developing analytical skills through different ways of using personal and professional **reflection** for learning and developing as a practitioner. The purpose of the book is to introduce you, the novice or more experienced practitioner, to different reflective models and frameworks, as well as ways of integrating personal and professional reflective insights to help support safe and effective practice. The aim is to assist you to develop a sense of agency in your own learning by broadening the scope and depth of your reflection to include biographical aspects. The reason for this is to help you to develop a life-wide (as well as a life-long) view of learning and reflection, which can sustain your practice and you as a practitioner.

This book should be seen as offering practical guidance to becoming reflective. It will be particularly useful for those starting out on such a process or wanting to try different methods. As you and your reflection develop, so too will your interests and reading include ever more complex concepts and professional experience. The chapters will encourage you to examine your experience and learning within the reflective process – through case studies, scenarios and activities that are rooted in the realities of practice and learning. This will help you to cope with the uncertainty of developing as a professional in a constructive way.

Chapter 1 sets the scene, showing how reflection has developed and its relevance for the new student and developing practitioner. It identifies potential benefits that reflection can bring for the person, profession, patients/clients, organisation and society. The chapter highlights the importance, for the novice and experienced practitioner, of recognising the significance of reflection for effective practice and the development of professional knowledge, particularly the fundamentals of practice.

Chapter 2 emphasises that learning not only takes place through formal courses or instruction but also extends into all areas of life. This chapter invites you to review some of these areas reflectively in order to extend learning potential. The focus here is on the types of knowledge produced through this reflective process, and the ways of knowing that can develop, which are crucial to life-long learning.

Chapter 3 introduces you, the student or developing practitioner, to autobiographical reflection as a means of helping to advance nursing knowledge in more diverse ways. In this chapter you are invited to integrate autobiographical reflection and learning with a sense of your developing identity, as well as to reflect on aspects of life that may reveal societal issues.

Chapter 4 introduces some of the wide range of reflective models and frameworks that you, as the student or practitioner, can draw upon when first starting to structure and frame your reflections. The chapter also considers the strengths and limitations of these, to help you to choose appropriately.

Chapter 5 introduces you, as the student or developing practitioner, to concepts of reflection as a transitional space in which you are encouraged to explore, develop and grow. As you progress, more will be expected in terms of knowledge, skills and decision-making. How a transitional space can draw out reflection and learning is a particular focus here.

Chapter 6 examines how student nurses and developing practitioners can influence their experiences, and how those experiences might influence them. It focuses on the role of reflexivity in developing opportunities for learning.

Chapter 7 invites you to cultivate a reflective approach to daily experience and integrate what you are learning. It is important for students to be able to acknowledge limitations within their knowledge as well as to own potential mistakes, and this chapter focuses on how to respond to fallibility – in yourself and in other professionals. This chapter introduces the concept of *mindfulness* and discusses its interface with reflection and reflexivity.

Chapter 8 considers how guided reflection, and reflecting with others, can deepen your understanding and analysis of situations, experiences and decisions, and offer support. The chapter also introduces ways of dealing with emotional residues of caring work.

Chapter 9 explores the purpose of reflective writing and introduces you, the student, to a variety of techniques. You are encouraged to try out some different exercises to help develop this skill. Some examples of reflective writing are discussed.

Chapter 10 looks at the possibilities new media offer for reflecting with others. It explores potential benefits and pitfalls and identifies how to develop your own digital story on which to reflect.

Chapter 11 emphasises the intense nature of critical reflection and its relevance to developing the skill of criticality. You are encouraged to consider your personal contributions and those of others to the development and outcomes of experiences.

## NMC's standards of proficiency for registered nurses

The Nursing and Midwifery Council (NMC) has standards of proficiency that must be met by applicants for entry onto different parts of the nursing and midwifery register. These standards are what the NMC deem as being necessary for the delivery of safe, effective nursing and midwifery practice.

This book includes the latest standards for 2018 onwards, taken from *Future Nurse: Standards of Proficiency for Registered Nurses* (NMC, 2018a).

## Learning features

Learning by reading text is not always easy. Therefore, to provide variety and assist with the development of independent learning skills, and the application of theory to practice, this book contains activities, example stories, scenarios (some with questions), case studies, concept summaries, further reading and useful websites to enable you to participate in your own learning. You will, however, need to develop your own study skills and 'learn how to learn' to get the best from the material. The book cannot provide all the answers but, rather, aims to provide a framework for your learning.

The activities in the book will help you to make sense of, and learn about, the material being presented. Some activities ask you to reflect on aspects of practice, or your experience of it, or the people or situations you encounter. *Reflection* is an essential skill in nursing, and it helps you to understand the world around you and often to identify how things might be improved. Other activities will help you develop key graduate skills such as your ability to *think critically* about a topic in order to challenge received wisdom, or your ability to *research a topic* and *find appropriate information and evidence* and to be able to make decisions using that evidence in situations that are often difficult and time pressured. Communication and working as part of a team are core to all nursing practice, and some activities will ask you to think about your *communication skills* to help develop these.

All the activities require you to take a break from reading the text, think through the issues presented and carry out some independent study, possibly using the internet. Where appropriate, there are sample answers presented at the end of each chapter, and these will help you to understand more fully your own reflections and independent study. You will gain most from the activities if you try to complete them yourself before reading the suggested answers. Remember, academic study will always require independent work; attending lectures will never be enough to be successful on your programme, and these activities will help to deepen your knowledge and understanding of the issues under scrutiny and give you practice at working on your own.

You might want to think about completing these activities as part of your personal development plan (PDP) or portfolio. After completing the activity, write it up in your PDP or portfolio in a section devoted to that particular skill, then look back overtime to see how far you have developed. You can also do more of the activities for a key skill in which you have identified a weakness; this will help build your skill and confidence in this area.

There is a glossary of terms at the end of the book, which provides an interpretation of some of the terminology in the context of the subject of the book; key terms are highlighted with bold text when first mentioned in the text.

All chapters have further reading and useful websites listed at the end, with notes to show you why we think they will be helpful to you. The websites will also help you to remain up to date with developments in this aspect of practice, as awareness of key issues grows and policies develop.

We hope that you find this book helpful in developing your professional practice and that it challenges you to ensure that you provide care and support that reduces the risk of vulnerability, and promotes dignity, respect and a positive quality of life. We wish you every success during your studies and beyond!

# Chapter 1 What is meant by reflection and reflective practice?

## NMC Future Nurse: Standards of Proficiency for Registered Nurses

This chapter will address the following platforms and proficiencies:

**Platform 1: Being an accountable professional**

1.3 Understand and apply the principles of courage, transparency and the professional duty of candour, recognising and reporting any situations, behaviours or errors that could result in poor care outcomes.

1.17 Take responsibility for continuous self-reflection, seeking and responding to support and feedback to develop their professional knowledge and skills.

**Platform 6: Improving safety and quality of care**

6.3 Comply with local and national frameworks, legislation and regulations for assessing, managing and reporting risks, ensuring the appropriate action is taken.

## Chapter aims

After reading this chapter you will be able to:

- define reflection and reflective practice;
- understand the relevance of reflection in nursing;
- identify benefits for the person, profession, patients/clients, organisations, and society;
- understand the requirements of the Nursing and Midwifery Council's Code (NMC, 2018b);

*(Continued)*

(Continued)

- understand the nature of accountability and reflection and how this relates to the 6 Cs of nursing;
- understand which legislation could impact on the nurse's role;
- begin to explore personal and professional forms of reflection.

## Case Study 1.1: Heather's reflection on professional practice

Heather was on a community-based learning disability nursing placement in the second year of her mental health nurse preparation programme. She enjoyed the placement, but found some aspects challenging, such as when an independent living resident became emotionally distressed. Heather's practice supervisor Barbara was often busy, and Heather frequently took her concerns home.

Yesterday Heather and Barbara visited 25-year-old Jack, who has a diagnosis of autism and had moved out of the family home to gain more independence. This was the first time that Barbara had met Jack because he had previously been under the care of another nurse, Mo. Barbara checked that Jack was coping with the change to his circumstances and that he had food in the house. Jack made Barbara and Heather a cup of tea and they talked about his week. During their discussion Jack spoke about Mo, saying he liked him a lot. He said that Mo had met him on Friday night when Jack was out with friends at the pub. Jack bought the drinks with his allowance, something Jack said he often did when Mo met him. After some further talk about other aspects of Jack's week, Barbara and Heather left.

On the way to the car Heather asked Barbara if it was acceptable for nurses to socialise with service users like Jack. Barbara said this was Mo's way of helping Jack assimilate into society and the local community and told Heather not to worry about it. She explained where they were going next and got in the car.

When Heather got home that evening, she could not stop thinking about her meeting with Jack and what Barbara had said. Heather tried to reflect on the situation but felt confused and unsure what to do. She was concerned that Mo had taken advantage of his position and behaved unprofessionally, allowing Jack to spend his allowance on him. Heather was also uneasy that Barbara did not appear concerned about this. Heather wondered whether this was because she was not yet fully aware of the policies and procedures used in the learning disability setting, or whether Barbara was covering for a colleague. Heather, therefore, felt she could not approach Barbara about her anxieties.

Heather, along with fellow mental health students, participated in an ongoing support group throughout the programme. She decided to discuss the issue with the group at the next session. The group was facilitated by Karim who asked her some reflective questions about what she was thinking and feeling, the evidence for this, and the alternatives and potential consequences of following these. Heather concluded that following the process for raising concerns about practice was the course of action she would take, with the help of her personal tutor.

# Introduction

As illustrated in Case Study 1.1, although we need to believe that healthcare professionals' intentions are honourable and that they do not mean to harm the people in their care, reports, unfortunately, suggest otherwise and we should be mindful of things that happen. A study among psychologists supporting service users with learning disability (Hewitt, 2014) suggests that 25 per cent of clients referred to psychology services reported some form of psychological, sexual and physical abuse, with 13 per cent of the perpetrators being staff. Those living with learning disability can have issues with physical and mental health and face problems when accessing healthcare. Research tells us that those living with a learning disability are dying prematurely. A high proportion of those deaths could have been treated or prevented (NHS England, 2025).

Professionals are sometimes fallible, especially now in our complicated healthcare landscape (Buckley, 2025). Case Study 1.1 is an illustration of how important reflection is to make sense of things and make morally effective decisions. The findings of the independent inquiry into the Mid Staffordshire National Health Service (NHS) Foundation Trust failings (Francis, 2013) highlight the potential consequences of ignoring concerns about care (see further reading at the end of the chapter). The report identified that patients' needs were ignored, that they were not treated with compassion and that when concerns were raised, they were not acted upon. In response to this indictment of care standards, the then Chief Nurse for England, Jane Cummins, in association with the Department of Health (2012), developed principles for care and compassion, described as the 6 Cs. More recent **Safeguarding Reviews,** such as, Whorlton Hall, conclude that a toxic and intimidating staff culture resulted in those most at risk having a lack of advocacy, indicating that compassionate care was seriously lacking to the detriment of vulnerable service users (Fish et al., 2023). Additionally, despite the Mid-Staffordshire report findings in 2013 Francis and Power (2023) believe that 'the current crisis in the NHS is a serious threat to patient safety and, it is clear that lives are being lost as a result... what we are witnessing across the NHS is the Mid Staffordshire scandal playing out on a national level.'

When reading Case Study 1.1 above, a number of thoughts may come to mind: 'Why did the practice supervisor find the contact between Mo and Jack acceptable?', 'Why did the student nurse not ask what the Trust policy was about socialising?', 'Why did the practice supervisor not ask what Heather's concerns were?' and 'What might have been done differently?' Even if reflection is not a familiar concept to you, particularly when starting your nurse preparation programme, this kind of curiosity and questioning forms the basis of personal reflection. This chapter sets the scene of what reflection is and its relevance for new students and more experienced practitioners. It contextualises reflection and **reflective practice** through tracing some of the main historical roots and key developments to help establish their importance in the nursing profession. Patient safety, accountability, responsibility, empathy, errors and near misses are examples of practice issues that can be influenced by reflection (or a lack thereof). This chapter further emphasises the significance of reflection for effective, professional practice and development of professional knowledge in accordance with legislation, the Nursing and Midwifery Council (NMC) Code (2018b) and the 6 Cs. The chapter concludes by considering accountability issues and the relationship to professional and personal forms of reflection. You are invited to complete a variety of activities and consider several case studies and scenarios. This will help you to start reflecting if you are a novice, or to develop reflection if you are a more experienced practitioner.

# What is reflection?

In the past decades, reflection has been defined in various ways: Dewey (1933) and Habermas (1971) suggest that reflection is a tool to be used in the development of knowledge. However, the outcome of reflection is different for the two theorists; Dewey considers reflection essential to *make sense of the world* and Habermas sees reflection as a means of *empowerment and political emancipation* (Moon, 2000, p. 15). These ideas then progress to thinking about our previous experience that helps develop **tacit knowledge** and **intuitive knowledge** (Johns & Freshwater, 2005). Experience and reflection become a continuous cycle in which our experiences are connected. This process changes us as individuals and strengthens our future actions (Gobbi, 2021). As nurses this process is a way to reach awareness of how and why things have occurred (Johns, 2025). Such reflection should be critical and focus on consistency and inconsistency of actual care delivery with values, standards and regulations (de Vries & Timmins, 2016).

Although formal definitions of reflection may seem academic and each appear to have a different focus, depending on the author and whether, they are speaking in generic terms (e.g., Dewey, Habermas and Moon) or within a specific nursing context (e.g., Johns and Freshwater) we should remember that reflection is not unusual. We carry it out in the car, on the train, while undertaking exercise and during and after conversations. Even deciding which washing powder or capsule to purchase is often a reflective process. In fact, wherever we have mental and physical space to think about things. Take some time out to think about what you did today and complete Activity 1.1.

## Activity 1.1 Reflection

Spend some time reviewing what you have done today. You should consider the whole day, note things that come to mind, prioritise them and answer the following questions:

- What things were significant and why?
- When and where did you find yourself thinking about something in more depth?
- Can you track changes to your thinking?
- What do you think about the issue now?

*There is an outline answer to this activity at the end of the chapter.*

When completing the activity, you may have identified another way that you could have done things, or things you might have said (or left unsaid), or you may arrive at a different conclusion. However, as a professional, this 'reflection' or 'thinking things over' will probably need to become more focused and structured to learn from the things we experience. Two important frameworks, the ***NMC Code (2018b)* and the *6 Cs*,** should inform the professional nurse's reflection and could be used to structure the reflective process (please refer to Chapter 4 for more information on reflective models).

Literature refers to 'tacit knowledge' as having a common understanding about something, whereas 'intuitive knowledge' means being sensitive to links with previous experience. In the example at the start of the chapter Heather is trying to make sense of things through reflecting on her own and with others to identify possible explanations for Mo's behaviour and the effects of that behaviour on Jack. Reflection is a way of examining your experience, explanations and alternative approaches to doing things. It may happen as part of an activity or later, when you have more time to think about what you have experienced. What is required is a curious mind that can accept the possibility of different explanations. Reflection means that thoughts about significant aspects of an experience are reconsidered and alternative explanations are contemplated. For the more experienced practitioner, reflection may reach greater depths because there is more knowledge and a wider range of experience to examine. For example, reflection may be triggered by a different response to a routine action and proceed beyond the immediate situation to consider knowledge, personal values and personal practice as well as the values and practice of others. When considering Heather's situation in Case Study 1.1, you might start the reflective process by considering the NMC Code (2018b). For Case Study 1.1, two sections of the NMC Code are particularly relevant: *Preserve safety* and *Promote professionalism and trust.* Take time to read the NMC Code, and you will find that the first section addresses raising concerns, and the second focuses on professional behaviour. Also relevant for this Case Study is to think about what legislation would be appropriate; for example, you might want to consider issues of safeguarding as identified in the Care Act 2014, the Safeguarding Vulnerable Groups Act 2006, the Mental Capacity Act 2005 and the Care Standards Act 2000. You could reflect on how the 6 Cs are demonstrated in care and professional practice currently. Perhaps consider that, although the 6 Cs form the value base for the nursing and midwifery professions the values of each practitioner rely on personal interpretation and experiences and could be conflicting (Buckley, 2025).

The 6 Cs are defined as shown in Figure 1.1.

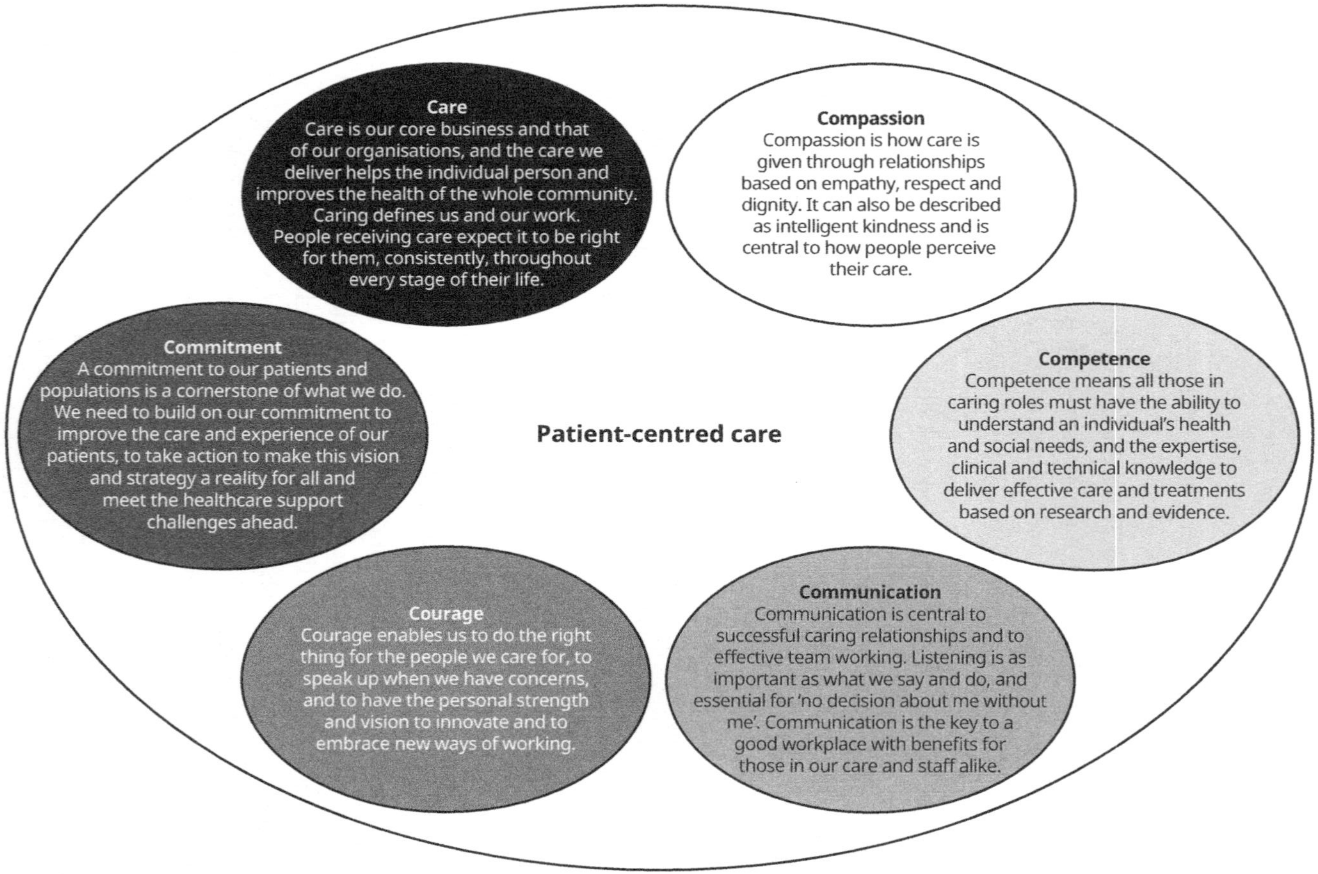


*Figure 1.1* The 6 Cs (from Department of Health and NHS Commissioning Board, 2012, p. 13)

You may want to think about Heather's need to have courage in taking this further. Why would this need courage? If you were in Heather's position, would you find it courageous to address the situation? Why would this be? You may have considered that Heather reflected on the way home and by sharing her concerns in the support group, and reflecting on them in more detail, consolidated her decision-making about what were the best options for Jack, for the organisation and for her. If you had been in Heather's situation, what would you think? Would you have raised this situation in the support group? Why? Try to identify explicitly what you think the problem is. In your opinion, how do you think the situation should or could be resolved? Now, attempt Activity 1.2, writing down your reflections as you work through it.

### Activity 1.2 Critical thinking

Read the example at the start of the chapter again and consider how/why reflection is relevant here. Write these points down. Now consider which legislation must be considered, and which elements of the NMC Code (2018b) and which of the 6 Cs are relevant to the case. Once you have considered and identified elements appropriate to the example, take this activity further by writing down why they are appropriate. Use the relevant documentation to support your ideas.

Read the following and make notes about courage and speaking up to help you with this activity.

Rafferty, A. M. & Leary, A. (2023). Nursing notes on a scandal. *Future Healthcare Journal, 10*(1), 3–6. https://doi-org.rcn.idm.oclc.org/10.7861/fhj.2023-FR102

*There is no outline answer at the end of the chapter for this individual activity*

Having worked through Activity 1.2, you may now think differently about Case Study 1.1. You may have found the situation overwhelming; but remain mindful that this is an opportunity to explore your personal values in relation to your professional and legal responsibilities. Working through these Case Studies, other explanations may need to be imagined (particularly for the inexperienced practitioner) and confirmed with someone more experienced. It is important to what you might like to happen from the reality of what is possible or likely; for example, imagining the potential reaction of a client or patient, or considering the possible consequences of a particular act. Please look at Scenario 1.1 and see if you can gain further understanding of the role of imagination in reflection. You are asked to identify some of these features after reading Scenario 1.1.

### Scenario 1.1: Biju

You are in your second year of my adult nurse preparation programme on the **Endoscopy** unit. You are working with your practice supervisor in the endoscopy theatre, assisting with a **colonoscopy** list. Your first patient is Biju, a 75-year-old man,

*(Continued)*

(Continued)

who is quite nervous. The documentation was checked to make sure you have the right patient, the correct preparation is completed and Biju has consented to the procedure. You are asked to reassure Biju while your supervisor inserts a cannula and starts to administer the prescribed sedative and **analgesia**.

The consultant calls you to look through the colonoscope at various stages, explaining the anatomy that you are observing. Towards the end of the procedure the consultant calls you over as they have found a lesion and suspect bowel cancer.

As you were present while Biju was being sedated your practice supervisor suggests it would help Biju to see a familiar face afterwards, so asks you to complete his aftercare.

The consultant comes to speak to Biju at the end of the morning. By this time Biju's daughter Bindu has arrived. You stay to observe the consultant telling Biju the bad news of suspected bowel cancer and what further processes would follow. You expect Biju and his daughter to become upset, but they remain remarkably calm. After the consultant is gone Biju and Bindu both smile and say it is 'karma'. Biju says he had had a good life, and this would help him in the next one.

Following Scenario 1.1, Activity 1.3 asks you to reflect on this experience.

### Activity 1.3 Reflection

- What might your responses be in such a situation?
- What have you learned whilst reflecting on this scenario?
- If you are an experienced nurse, how might your reflective imagination have differed from those of a student nurse or a preceptorship nurse?

*There are outline answers to these questions at the end of the chapter.*

Having read Scenario 1.1 and answered the questions at the end, you may see that reflection using imagination can identify several different strands of a situation, and how this may be relevant to practice. We return to the role of imagination in reflection in Chapter 3. Scenario 1.1 also illustrates the importance of reflecting on events.

The chapter now proceeds to define reflective practice.

# What is reflective practice?

In addition to the definitions of reflection indicated at the start of this chapter, Rolfe (2011) suggests that reflective practice is a process that develops understanding of what it means to be a practitioner, and Jasper (2003) suggests that it links theory and practice through the practitioner consciously thinking through the experience. This is an important activity for novice practitioners to help develop an understanding of their role and support the learning of new skills. Reflection can occur within the experience or by looking back at the experience. Schön (1991) identifies these as reflection-in-action and reflection-on-action. Thinking about things requires knowledge of theory to develop answers, but theory needs to be mapped on to a situation if we are to use it for problem-solving. Reflection-in-action refers to knowing what to do and making a difference within a given situation – in Case Study 1.1, Heather identified a situation 'in-the-moment' and attempted to address it, but, due to lack of knowledge or confidence, she was not able to follow it through. Reflection-on-action, however, means examining some of those 'in-the-moment' decisions for the possibility of other choices and ways of acting, and how these insights might shape and develop future practice. This happens after the situation, just as Heather had thought about the situation of Jack and Mo in the evening once she was home. Besides questioning the Jack/Mo situation, Heather could have thought about why she was not able to press the discussion with Barbara, and what she could have done differently to address her questions or misgivings more satisfactorily in the future. Reflection often contains multiple levels of exploration. As seen from Case Study 1.1, Heather reflected on the actual situation and whether the contact between Jack and Mo was professional. However, at a more personal level she could reflect on how she had discussed her reservations with Barbara and how she could have done this differently. This is where the courage C and the communication C from the 6 Cs can be explained. Did Heather feel intimidated because of her lack of knowledge about policy? Perhaps she felt uncomfortable raising questions of professional practice about a colleague with whom she had regularly worked? These elements of reflection are more personal, lead to professional growth and are discussed in later chapters.

At this point we move from reflection-in-action and reflection-on-action to focus more on problem-solving, which can take the form of rational thinking based on protocols and procedures. However, imitating role-modelled behaviour in dealing with situations is a form of non-reflective learning (Jarvis, 2006). For example, when undertaking a drug round, if the practitioner is mainly intent on fulfilling the requirements of the seven rights of drug administration, through checking the right dose, right drug, right patient, right time and right route, right documentation, right reason and does not reflectively consider their actions, knowledge or the patient, this does not develop learning. What aids learning is looking beyond the basic actions to examine understanding and personal responses. Reflective practice requires careful consideration of knowledge and ideas. This is described as 'reflection-before-action' and 'reflection-beyond-action' (Edwards, 2017).

As illustrated above, reflective practice considers practice as a whole, consisting of different layers and elements that cannot always be rationalised. Individuals are unique, and human factors may be uncertain, even messy. Reflective practice is, therefore, based on experience and intuitive learning of which you may be unaware until you need to respond to a situation. It may seem easier for some practitioners to respond to situations because they have greater experience to draw on, but reflection always takes courage and commitment. Reflecting on practice helps you become more aware of your learning, which is crucial for developing skills and competence at any career stage. This becomes equally as important when considering what happens in practice, such as having learned the evidence-based hand-washing technique, and successfully passing the related assessments (**espoused theories**), but then taking shortcuts in the busyness of a shift, using the full technique only after what you consider to be 'dirty' procedures (**theories in use).** This practice, although incorrect, might be wrongly perceived as 'acceptable' and is clearly not using the taught theories of safe care (Geltmeyer et al., 2025).

By using critical reflection, we can become aware of such discrepancies in our own actions, re-evaluate the quality of our work and develop alternative behaviour. This is why courage and commitment, as mentioned earlier, are important as critical reflection can be an uncomfortable process, in which individuals become aware of and confront previously unconscious qualities, behaviour or tendencies in themselves that can be distressing. In this way reflective practice can contribute to organisational learning through its members (Barchard, 2022).

Critical reflection can be taken even further. Knowledge derived from practice does not add to professional knowledge unless it has been reflected on for its significance (Sherwood, 2024). For example, as a novice practitioner you may have worked with healthcare assistants and your practice supervisor. You may have been involved in completing a care element, such as a bed bath, with both at some point. You may have noticed differences in how the care was completed. However, unless you reflect on this and reach conclusions about the significance of the differences, the care will remain a task that was completed in different ways, and perhaps not the expression of nursing knowledge and values that it might have been. The learning and articulation of values embedded within this episode of care will be lost. Equally, an experienced practitioner who may have to complete similar tasks can gain greater insight and knowledge through reflecting on how each episode of care might be the same and yet different each time they are performed, and what knowledge and values are being used and maybe even generated, in order to avoid simple repetition of experience that does not constitute learning.

Looking at the definitions of reflection earlier in this chapter, you notice they all promote learning in some way. Deconstructing your practice experience brings us to another learning theory; namely that of David Kolb (1984). In his theory he describes four **learning styles**.

As we can see from Figure 1.2, there are reflective and practical stages where, according to Kolb and Kolb (2013), optimal learning takes place by continually working through both the practical and reflective 'modes'. From this you can see that learning is an ongoing spiral process that provides you with more depth of understanding and/or increasing capability as you progress.

Now apply some of the principles of reflective practice to your own practice by completing Activity 1.4.

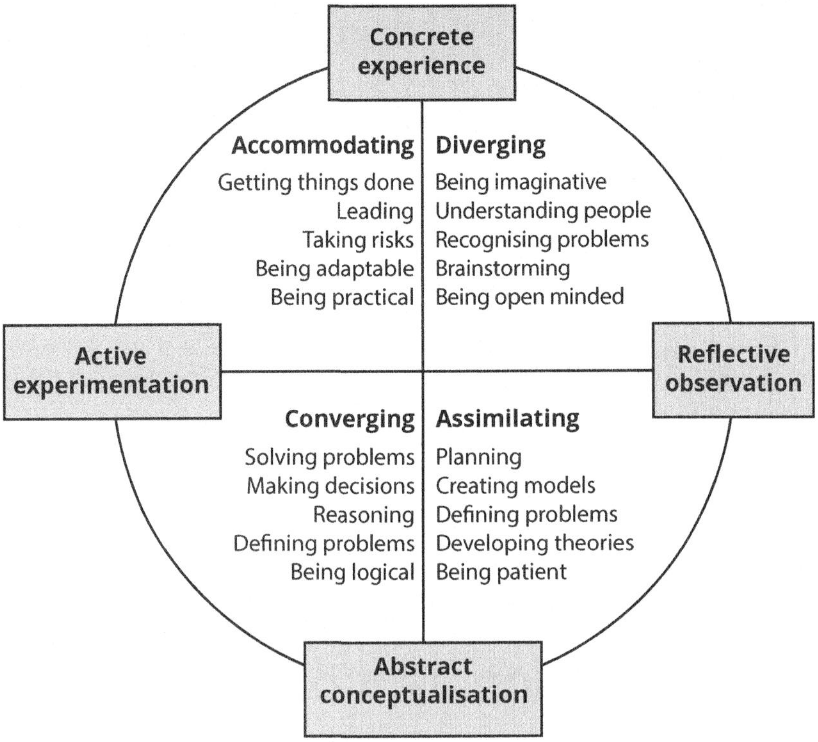


*Figure 1.2* Kolb's learning cycle (adapted from Kolb and Kolb, 2013, p. 8)

## Activity 1.4 Critical thinking

**When you are next in practice and in a nursing situation, try to consider the following:**

- What is going on?
- What knowledge are you using?
- Which values are you drawing upon and articulating in the situation?
- What decisions are you making?
- How have you come to those decisions?
- Are you trying out different things?
- What is changing your thinking, if anything?
- How are the above relevant to the 6 Cs?

*Allow an interval of at least a day between the situation and reflecting on it further. Now ask yourself the same questions again.*

- Have your answers changed and, if so, how?
- What learning are you taking from this?

*(Continued)*

(Continued)

*It is useful to keep asking yourself these questions, maintaining a reflective diary to track your learning and development.*

It may help to document this activity by using the pro forma offered at the end of the chapter.

There are outline answers to these questions at the end of the chapter.

As a second activity, using the same situation that you used for the exercise above, work through Kolb's reflective cycle, making a note of where you start in the process. See the notes at the end of the chapter for this exercise.

Chapter 7 addresses the theme of reflective practice again by looking at what constitutes the reflective practitioner. Having defined reflection and reflective practice, this chapter now looks at the development of reflection and its relevance in the context of nursing.

# History and development of reflection in the context of nursing

It may be assumed that pioneers of nursing (such as Florence Nightingale) came to different conclusions about what was needed in terms of sanitation in hospitals, through reflecting on the problem; this is illustrated in the preface to *Notes on Nursing: What it is and What it is Not* (Nightingale, 1969). Nightingale states: *Every day sanitary knowledge, or the knowledge of nursing, or in other words, of how to put the constitution in such a state that it will have no disease, or that it can recover from disease, takes a higher place* (Nightingale, 1969). One could argue that Nightingale's interpretation of sanitary fits with Jasper's (2003) concept of reflection linking theory and practice through conscious thought and Rolfe's (2011) idea that reflective practice is a process that develops understanding of what it means to be a practitioner. What is clear is that possibilities for reflection appear in nursing through research studies that explore different types of nursing knowledge. For example, Carper (1978) identified patterns of knowing that looked further than a medical model of disease management to where nurses discovered new nursing theories through working out their ideas. Benner's (1984) influential work explained how nurses developed their knowledge in practice, and Watson (1988, 2008) recognised the importance of previous practice in shaping nurses' perceptions of knowledge and urged nurses to develop new insights. Schön (1991) suggested reflection as getting to the heart of how professionals think in action. Moon's (2000) work *Reflection in Learning and Professional Development* is a worthwhile read to obtain a more detailed history of reflection and its development.

Changes in nursing education have meant that there has been increasing focus on reflection as a tool for teaching and learning. Since the early 1990s, interest in reflection and its contribution within nurse education has grown (Pierson, 1998). In 1994, nursing's regulatory body at the time pronounced that all nurses needed to maintain a portfolio of evidence of learning activity and listed reflection as an essential component of this activity (UKCC, 1994). This requirement has been updated by the NMC (NMC, 2017), which states that reflection on the outcome of any type of learning is essential for maintaining knowledge, skills and competence as a nurse, incorporating it into the NMC revalidation process. It is evident that decision-making skills are essential in the preparation and education of nurses (NMC, 2024; Willis, 2015). Reflection helps with this by examining evidence and alternative courses of action, thereby coming to an informed decision. Thus reflection, in the context of nursing, is a foundation for learning that takes place both inside and outside the classroom.

Discourse between novice and experienced practitioners is part of an ongoing reflective dialogue that continues to take nursing practice forward through new insights that are revealed within such discussions (Johns, 2012). Thus, the student nurse and the experienced practice supervisor can contribute to nursing knowledge in dynamic ways through interaction. For example, questioning and exploring what is known about a situation or topic also bring what is unknown into view and both can be considered as part of developing a wider understanding as well as critically considering what values are brought to bear on a situation and why. This is important to develop the profession, as you can see from the following dialogue between a student and practice supervisor.

## Student and practice supervisor dialogue

| | |
|---|---|
| Student: | *I have never come across anyone with a learning disability. How do I talk to them?* |
| Practice supervisor: | *How do you like to be talked to?* |
| Student: | *I like people to use my first name and for us to share our views on the topic of conversation.* |
| Practice supervisor: | *That is a good way to talk to someone. Ask them to tell you a bit about themselves and share their views. What have you learned about communication in your preparation programme?* |
| Student: | *We have learned about how to build therapeutic relationships using verbal and non-verbal communication and about empathy and using the 6 Cs. But I am not sure how they might respond.* |
| Practice supervisor: | *We don't know how anyone might respond – we have to take our cues from them. What is your main concern?* |
| Student: | *That I might upset them and not know what to do.* |
| Practice supervisor: | *One way of avoiding this is to learn to read emotional cues or what is sometimes called 'emotional intelligence'. If you attune yourself to others' emotional cues, you can start to work out how they are feeling and responding to what you are saying. When I started nursing, I found it hard to talk to people because I was very shy. I am still shy, but what has helped me is learning to move beyond my own feelings by becoming aware of others' feelings and responding accordingly. This is part of emotional intelligence.* |
| Student: | *I think we had a lecture about emotional intelligence and watched a video about empathy.* |
| Practice supervisor: | *Start talking to one of our residents today by finding out a bit about each other. You could start by saying what your interests are and ask them about theirs. Then revisit your notes from that lecture and reflect on what you have learned today. We will discuss your reflection about this tomorrow.* |

The student and practice supervisor dialogue illustrates how thinking about and reflecting on practice issues are important ways for professional knowledge to develop. 'Socratic questioning', which asks for thinking, is an essential part of this learning process. The idea of developing understanding and knowledge of nursing through reflection brings benefits for the nurse and patient. Some of these benefits are explored in the next section.

# Benefits of reflection

Reflection can help us affirm actions but can also trigger us to consider correcting other actions. It may enable us to translate successful strategies into new situations and thus continue to develop them. Equally, when reflection reveals problems with an action taken, it enables you to avoid using that action in similar circumstances or allows you to consider other corrections. It can help you to identify the causes of errors or potential errors, called near misses, thereby promoting patient safety and learning as recommended in the Francis report (2013). From this perspective, reflection can help raise your confidence in your abilities and highlight things to avoid. Some benefits from reflection for the individual practitioner, the organisation and the patient are summarised in Figure 1.3.

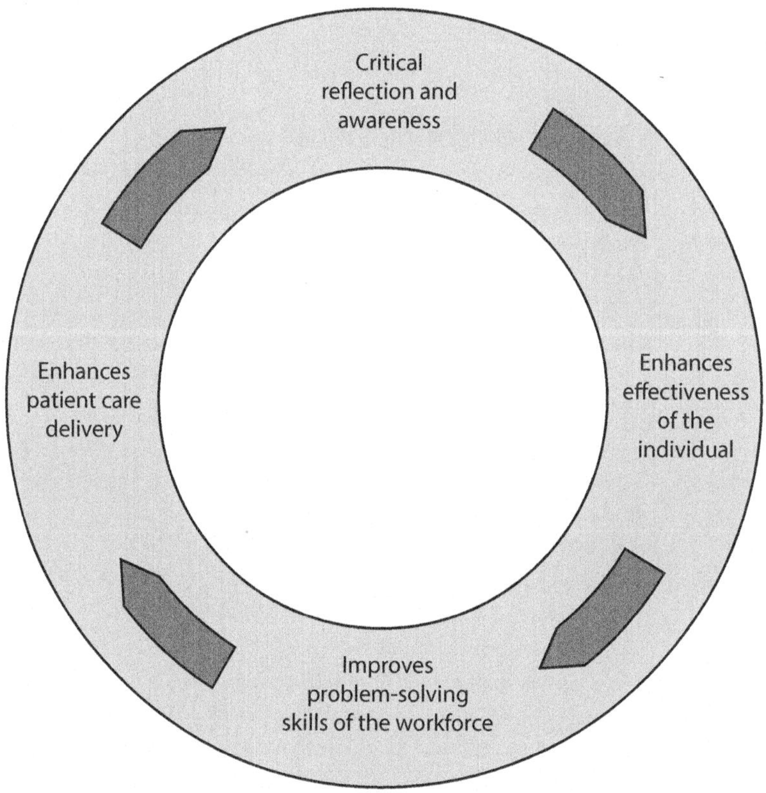


*Figure 1.3* Benefits from reflection for the individual practitioner, the organisation and the patient

Reflection means making the familiar unfamiliar, the unfamiliar familiar or looking at situations with fresh eyes and a curious enquiry (Voldbjerg et al., 2021). You will be able to chart the development of your effectiveness in problem-solving and delivering patient care by using reflection throughout your nursing programme. Equally, as an experienced practitioner, reflection helps you re-evaluate your personal effectiveness in problem-solving and managing patient care. The organisation benefits from individuals improving their skills, as do the clients and patients using the service. Therefore, reflection as practised by you would reflect across the profession throughout your career. Complete Activity 1.5, in which you consider in more detail some of the benefits of reflection.

### Activity 1.5 Reflection

As a student nurse you will need to learn clinical skills. Think about the first skill you learned.

- What were the highlights of learning this skill?
- What were the problems?
- How did you deal with any existing or potential problems?
- How did you feel about learning the skill at the time?
- How did you feel about putting it into practice with a real person for the first time?
- Did your practice change in the live setting and, if so, why?
- What do you think about your practice of the skill now, after reflecting on it through these questions?
- What learning are you taking forward from this?

If you are an experienced practitioner, consider the same questions in relation to decision-making and management skills.

*There is an outline answer to this activity at the end of the chapter.*

Once you have identified your learning of a skill through Activity 1.5 and your evaluation of it, you will have a clearer picture of your knowledge and ability. These are important aspects of your personal responsibility and accountability. We now move on to consider how accountability relates to reflection.

## Accountability and reflection

The NMC Code expects nurses and midwives to maintain their knowledge in order to provide safe and effective practice (NMC, 2018b). Working within the boundaries of the NMC Code is part of the standard of professional behaviour expected of nurses and nursing practice. As suggested earlier, simply receiving new ideas does not translate into becoming knowledgeable. Reflection is needed to take new concepts and understand how to use them. Therefore, if you are expected to maintain your knowledge, it follows that thinking and reflecting on that knowledge and what you do are part of your accountability as a nurse. Case Studies 1.2 and 1.3 look at Mandy's responsibility and Sarah's accountability as a way of illustrating the process of reflecting on these aspects within learning from practice.

## Case study 1.2: Mandy's responsibility

Mandy was in the second year of her nursing programme. She had been working in a day surgery unit that encompassed a pre-assessment area, ward and theatre suite, with the ward phone as the central contact point. The unit was busy with people coming and going, the phone ringing with relatives enquiring about patient discharges or doctors asking for information. In one such phone call, a doctor asked Mandy to pass a message to the theatre staff about a certain instrument that should be available for the afternoon theatre list. Unfortunately, Mandy was distracted by a patient who started vomiting and needed her assistance, and she forgot to pass the message on.

When the afternoon began, a very upset nurse rang from the theatre suite to ask why the message about the specific instrument had not been passed on. The patient's procedure had to be cancelled because the instrument could not be prepared in time.

The doctor came to apologise to the patient who was very unhappy. The theatre staff were upset that they appeared inefficient. The ward manager wanted to know who had taken the message and not passed it on. Mandy was also upset when she realised it was her and thought what to do next.

## Activity 1.6 Reflection

- If you were Mandy, what would you think about, what would you reflect on and what would be your response?
- How does Case Study 1.2 relate to the 6 Cs?

*There are outline answers to these questions at the end of the chapter.*

Now consider another day in Mandy's placement, on the same unit. After reading Case Study 1.3 and Activity 1.7, now identify what aspects you might need to reflect on and what your learning might be.

## Case Study 1.3: Whose accountability?

Mandy was working a shift on day surgery with her practice supervisor, Sarah. It was a Friday and the patients who had recovered from their procedures were eager to go home. Mandy was preparing Judy, who had undergone a **haemorrhoidectomy**, for discharge. Haemorrhoidectomy can be a painful procedure, and Judy was being discharged with prescribed analgesia. The form of this analgesia was contraindicated in people who had asthma because it could induce an asthmatic episode. As Mandy was checking the medication and talking to Judy, she realised that there was a history of asthma, although Judy did not take regular medication for it. Nevertheless, Mandy brought this to the attention of her practice supervisor, explaining that the drug had been prescribed and what she had found out about its contraindications. She reflected on what might have happened if she had not noticed. Would she have been responsible, as in the previous episode? Who would be accountable if the Judy did subsequently experience an asthmatic episode at home?

### Activity 1.7 Reflection

- If you were Mandy, what would you reflect on in this situation?
- If you were Sarah, what would you reflect on in this situation? (If you are a novice practitioner, leave this part of the question.)
- How are responsibility and accountability assigned in Case Study 1.3?
- What might Mandy have learned from this situation?
- What might Sarah have learned from this situation? (If you are a novice practitioner, leave this part of the question.)

*There are outline answers to these questions at the end of the chapter.*

Case Study 1.3 and Activity 1.7 may have helped give you a clearer idea of some of the differences between responsibility and accountability, and the role of reflection in helping to make sense of this. However, it is important to note that responsibility and accountability go hand in hand and, although the two are separated in the examples above, we are accountable for our actions. This is especially important when undertaking your nursing programme because it can sometimes appear less clear in practice. Equally, as an experienced practitioner, reflecting on near-miss situations is important for adjusting practice. The chapter now looks at personal and professional forms of reflection that can help with this.

## Personal and professional forms of reflection

Journal writing is one method of developing reflective learning (Alt et al., 2022). The private log, or blog, has become a popular way of identifying what has been learned. This is usually private and only enters the public domain when shared in a progress review or to inform assignment content. This forms part of a portfolio to evidence learning. Students on a nurse preparation programme may be asked to enter reflections on learning into an online **e-portfolio**, for example, PebblePad, with different templates such as structured reflection, a blog and curriculum vitae (CV) assigned to different aspects of the programme. The tutor can view the information only when this is shared by the student. The issue of using digital media for reflection is explored in more detail in Chapter 10. During your preparation programme you will have been asked to reflect on a variety of situations and Case Studies, in the same way as you are in this book. You may be asked to reflect on your assignments in the form of case studies, where you might include a review of your actions and contribution to the patient's care. Complete Activity 1.8 as a way of starting to think about recording your reflective learning. The issue of reflective writing is explored in more detail in Chapter 9.

## Activity 1.8 Documenting reflection

Think about the main elements of your nursing programme. Write a reflection on your progress in each of these areas.

If you are an experienced practitioner, think about the main elements of your career development and write a reflection on your progress.

*There is an outline answer to this activity at the end of the chapter.*

For the experienced practitioner, reflection involves thinking about the nursing identity and reconstructing experience in order to identify how to progress. As a novice to nursing, you develop your own professional identity through undertaking the same process and this type of reflection examines aspects such as confidence, goal-setting, positivity, relationships, acceptance, loss and persistence (Artioli et al., 2021).

For example, nursing a dying patient may call into question our own mortality. Reconstructing the experience by looking at how we deal with loss might offer a way of examining how loss is interpreted in the context of dying and of others' experience. This may stimulate reflective thinking about possible courses of action for helping others to face loss. Reflective writing may be entered into a private diary and considered privately during such 'working out'. Professional forms of reflection may take place individually or in a group through a variety of ways, such as clinical supervision or action learning. Different forms of reflecting with others are explored in greater detail in Chapter 8.

## Chapter summary

This chapter has introduced reflection and reflective practice and some of the contemporary drivers of why reflection is important for nursing practice. Offering activities that ask the novice and developing nurse to review thinking and practice provides an opportunity to start developing reflection in relation to safe and effective nursing practice and decision-making. The examples help to illustrate the benefits of reflection and the relationship between accountability and reflection, encouraging you to start considering how this is relevant to your learning and practice, working within a regulatory code. Different forms of reflection and reflective practice are explained in later chapters.

## Brief outline answers

In this section, answers to the chapter's activities will be outlined and explained.

### Activity 1.1 Reflection

Your answer might have considered:

- getting up;
- interaction with others at home;
- travelling to work;
- priorities for work;
- completing work;
- coming home.

When thinking about which aspects were significant and why, you may have first been alerted by triggered emotions, for example, anxiety, satisfaction or anger, which led you to consider the trigger; this might have been a decision that you had made or were finding difficult to make. From here you can then re-evaluate the situation.

## Activity 1.2 Critical thinking

In the example, you might note that Heather is using courage, commitment, and communication within the case to safeguard Jack's interests. The role of reflection has been to make sense of her feelings and then to objectively evaluate her options. The fact that she is feeling uncomfortable about the situation with Jack and Mo is a cue to explore the situation more fully. Jack is a vulnerable adult and one of Heather's considerations is to explore what legislation says about safeguarding (you might want to look the Care Act 2014, the Safeguarding Vulnerable Groups Act 2006, the Mental Capacity Act 2005 and the Care Standards Act 2000). The Acts are in agreement regarding the carer's responsibility to protect the service user's interests. The 2021 National Institute for Health and Care Excellence (NICE) guideline, *Autism Spectrum Disorder in Adults: Diagnosis and Management*, recommends that healthcare professionals provide activities that promote social integration and minimise isolation. One could, therefore, argue that Mo's intentions of going with Jack to the bar aligns with this, but it is not considered professional conduct. According to the NMC's Code (2018b), sections on promoting professionalism (specifically items 20.1, 20.5, 20.6, 20.8, and 21.1), taking advantage of a service user, adhering to professional boundaries and accepting gifts, are considered to be serious issues of professional conduct. Heather is obliged to escalate her concerns according to the NMC's Code sections about preserving safety (specifically items 16.1, 16.3, 17.1, 17.2, and 17.3) (NMC, 2018b). As Barbara did not seem particularly concerned, when Heather talked to her, the responsibility is still with Heather to consider next steps. As a student, Heather would have access to an escalating concerns policy and would be strongly advised to discuss the situation with her personal tutor or the liaison lecturer for the practice area.

## Activity 1.3 Reflection

The significant features in Scenario 1.1 that you have likely reflected on are:

- the breaking of bad news;
- The persons' reaction;
- Your knowledge of other religions and cultures.

Did you use imagination to consider aspects where you did not have knowledge, namely:

- the service users reaction to bad news;
- how you would respond if you were asked what the result of the procedure was;
- what happens next;
- the consequences of any lack of knowledge about other religions and cultures.

Were there any additional features that you reflected on whilst imagining you were in this position?

As an experienced nurse your reflective imagination might have differed from those of a student nurse by identifying the significant features as:

- your accountability in this situation;
- how to offer additional support without causing offence.

You might have used imagination to consider the aspects you did not have knowledge of, such as:

- how the family might react to change;
- whether you have sufficient knowledge of other cultures and religions to understand your patient's response.

Although this activity is, fundamentally, about developing awareness of your own strengths and limitations, there are several items from the NMC's Code (2018b) that underpin this activity. It is worth considering these; for example, Section 2 *Prioritise people* (items 2.1, 2.2, 2.3, 2.4, and 2.6), which accentuates the need for partnership working and the role of the professional to empower service users to take responsibility for their own health and well-being, and 20.7 of Section 20, which calls for professionals not to express their own personal beliefs.

## Activity 1.4 Critical thinking

The second activity, using the same nursing situation that you used for the reflective activity, works through Kolb's **reflective cycle**. For example:

- Start by reflecting on the actual experience of the situation and the physical 'doing' that was involved; this means that you would start at the top of the cycle 'Concrete experience'. It is helpful to jot down in bullet points what you did.
- Then, look back at the experience by thinking about it and reviewing how things went; so, you would commence the cycle with 'Reflective observation'. Now is the time to think about how it felt and whether things went according to plan (what went well, and which elements were challenging). Again, make notes for each of the bullet points that you noted under 'Concrete experience'.
- In the next step you consider what you have learned from the experience and, in doing so, you would be engaging with 'Abstract conceptualisation'. At this stage, identify which point(s) you want to focus on and note why you want to focus on these points (often this relates to something that worked out differently to your expectations or an element of the activity that you feel uncertain about). Ask yourself why these points are important and try to find answers for yourself. Think of sources such as NICE guidelines, the NMC Code (2018b), *British National Formulary* (BNF) and theoretical sources such as textbooks, online packages, etc.
- The final step is to plan how you would approach the situation/activity the next time, planning for 'Active experimentation'.

Clearly, the next time you undertake the activity you would start your learning process at the 'Active experimentation' stage and work through the cycle from that point.

## Activity 1.5 Reflection

You may have thought about nursing skills such as taking a pulse and blood pressure: the difficulty of hearing the blood pressure when taking a manual measurement and of being nervous when faced with a real patient. As your skill develops you may have identified subtle nuances, such as a slight variation in where the brachial artery might be located in different patients. You may have learned that a manual measurement is often more accurate than an electronic one when blood pressure is significantly abnormal.

As an experienced practitioner you may have thought about decision-making in relation to problem-solving, planning and implementing care. As your skill develops you may have identified that you can do this quickly while dealing with competing demands. You may consider management skills such as allocating the skill mix of staff and liaising with the hierarchy of management. You may have learned the strengths and weaknesses of your interpersonal skills and management strategies.

## Activity 1.6 Reflection

In this Case Study, Mandy might think about talking to the doctor and theatre staff to take responsibility for the omission. She is likely to reflect on the circumstances that led her to forget and what she might have done differently, and how to avoid the omission in the future. Her initial response was to get upset when confronted by the ward manager, but thereafter she might have regained her confidence from having thought things through and reflecting on how to do things differently. The most relevant principle from the 6 Cs is communication.

## Activity 1.7 Reflection

In this Case Study, Mandy might reflect on what led her to identify the near miss. Sarah might reflect on the assessment of the patient, interprofessional communication, pharmacological knowledge and patient collaboration in care planning. In this Case Study, Mandy was responsible for completing the delegated task of preparing the patient for discharge and reporting new information or concerns. Sarah was accountable for acting on that information and for overseeing the care Mandy gave to the patient, including any drugs to take home. Mandy is likely to have learned that she has good assessment and observation skills which helped her to check information appropriately. Sarah might have learned that, no matter how experienced, professionals are fallible. She may also have learned that students can help to interrogate practice. When reflecting on Mandy's situation, it would be advisable to consider how this relates to the NMC Code (2018b); for example, the section *Practise effectively* (items 8.1, 8.2, 8.3, 8.4, 8.5, and 8.6), which relates to sharing information and appropriate communication between team members.

## Activity 1.8 Documenting reflection

You might have written reflections on:

- developing graduate skills;
- knowledge and proficiency with information technology;
- developing essential clinical skills;
- practice;
- personal development planning.

As an experienced practitioner you might have written reflections on:

- developing leadership and management skills;
- developing your knowledge and proficiency in different practice situations;
- dealing with conflict and change.

To help document some of the reflection that you may have undertaken in completing the activities in this chapter, you might want to consider:

- description of experience;
- evaluation;
- analysis;
- future action.

The following pro forma is offered to help you begin to document reflection.

| **Pro forma for documenting reflection** |
|---|
| Self-assessing experience: |
| Main points identified from reflection on the experience: |
| **Pro forma for documenting reflection** |
| Learning points: |
| How will this learning be applied in the future? |
| Professional development achieved? |

## Further reading

**Delves-Yates, C.** (2018). *Essential clinical skills for nurses: Step by step* (2nd ed.). Sage.

This book offers a step-by-step approach to developing clinical skills in any field.

**Delves-Yates, C.** (2025). *Beginner's guide to reflective practice in nursing* (2nd ed.). Sage.

This book is specifically for nursing students and trainee nursing associates to assist you to succeed in your studies and practice.

**Francis, R.** (2013). *Report of the mid staffordshire NHS foundation trust public inquiry: Executive summary.* HMSO. www.midstaffspublicinquiry.com/sites/default/files/report/Executive%20summary.pdf

This report identifies the full scale of the deficits and failings in care and offers recommendations for how these might be avoided in the future. You may like to relate your reading to your own practice and reflect on what further action to take.

**Seedhouse, D.** (2020). *Using personal judgement in nursing and healthcare.* Sage.

This book assists you to pose questions, which may have occurred to you throughout this chapter. Such as, what is personal judgement? How can it help me interpret and follow official guidelines? How can I use it successfully in my daily practice?

## Useful websites

**https://www.autism.org.uk/advice-and-guidance/professional-practice?page=1**

This professional resource has monthly updates by professionals and autistic people sharing knowledge, good practice, research and advice for anyone working with autistic people.

**https://www.businessballs.com/freepdfmaterials/reflective-practice-self-assessment.pdf**

This website offers useful resources to help the reader to reflect. You are invited to try out the 'How reflective are you?' self-assessment.

**https://www.england.nhs.uk/long-read/guidance-to-support-implementation-of-the-mental-capacity-act-in-acute-trusts-for-adults-with-a-learning-disability/**

This resource provides practical tools and resources to assist the understanding and application of the Mental Capacity Act 2005.

# Chapter 2 Life-wide, life-long, and life-deep learning and reflection

## NMC Future Nurse: Standards of Proficiency for Registered Nurses

This chapter will address the following platforms and proficiencies:

**Platform 1: Being an accountable professional**

1.8 Demonstrate the knowledge, skills, and ability to think critically when applying evidence and drawing on experience to make evidence-informed decisions in all situations.

1.17 Take responsibility for continuous self-reflection, seeking and responding to support and feedback to develop their professional knowledge and skills.

**Platform 2: Promoting health and preventing ill health**

2.12 Protect health through understanding and applying the principles of infection prevention and control, including communicable disease surveillance and antimicrobial stewardship and resistance.

## Chapter aims

By the end of this chapter, you will be able to:

- define what is meant by life-wide, life-long, and life-deep learning;
- identify the breadth of knowledge that a nurse needs to ensure is current;
- identify some of the contexts in which learning takes place;
- identify features of learning in formal and less formal ways;
- consider types of knowledge and ways of knowing;
- understand how the person learns through reflection.

### Case Study 2.1: Experience of sharing knowledge

Omar had completed his first placement in the second year of the adult nursing programme and was undertaking the next module about acute care. The focus of the session was on the importance of accurate assessment and the students were asked to investigate a variety of assessment tools which encompassed multiple body systems. The scenarios presented surgical, medical, and emergency situations allowing the class to apply some of these assessment strategies and techniques.

Omar's placement had been in radiology where he had seen **robotic-assisted procedures** for **prostatectomies** and **myomectomies** which offered less invasive and more straightforward surgery. Omar reflected on the importance of accurate observation for these patients and realised that the assessment tools under discussion were applicable and could be used in different environments, with some groups of patients; the procedures still represented acute care because the patient was sedated and vulnerable to complications. Omar discussed these scenarios with his peers during the group work and, together, they applied the assessment strategies.

Feeding the group work back to the rest of the class, Omar offered the radiology scenarios to illustrate their application of the assessment tools and problem-solving, illustrating that the assessment tools were useable in different environments where people were exposed to acute episodes within care. The tutor asked Omar to explain more about the procedures to expand the knowledge of the whole class and her own, because she was not as familiar with robotic procedures.

Reflecting later, Omar realised that no matter how knowledgeable a person may be, learning does not stop with a qualification. Through explaining his understanding of the procedures to the class, Omar was also able to identify gaps in his knowledge in terms of the available assessment strategies and tools.

## Introduction

Learning is often multidimensional in terms of where and how it takes place. Looking at the outcome skills suggested at the start of this chapter, it is clear that developing and maintaining knowledge are not limited to clinical settings and patient or service user issues. As illustrated in Case Study 2.1 knowledge needs to be current in relation to developments in policy and guidelines, technology and political and health economic landscapes. Yet, learning is also a very individual process and what is carried forward may only be gauged by the individual. What is grasped may not always be what is taught. In Case Study 2.1, what is grasped is the need to assert a knowledge base, even if this differs from the examples being taught. The quality of the response received may influence whether this learning is taken forward or inhibited. To take ownership of learning requires understanding of where and how learning can take place.

This chapter emphasises that learning not only takes place through formal courses or instruction, but extends into all areas of life, a theme that is taken forward in Chapter 3. This chapter defines what is meant by life-wide, life-long, and life-deep learning and offers an example of each. We explore the contexts in which nurses might learn and consider them in terms of their levels of formality and learners' autonomy to design aspects of their own learning. At this point, it is important to accentuate the importance of taking responsibility for your own learning process and, wherever possible, being proactive in creating a learning environment. The chapter identifies different types of knowledge, how nurses come to know and how this relates to reflection. It concludes by summarising the interrelationship of reflection, developing an evidence base and informal learning.

Throughout the chapter, you are invited to complete activities and consider case studies and scenarios that enable you to examine the different contexts of your learning and analyse the progression of your learning.

# What is life-wide learning?

Life-wide learning is learning that is not limited to the classroom but that extends into other areas of life. This form of learning is broad and includes how we learn to be resilient and manage challenges and adversity (Boyd, 2023). Experience from these real-life situations allows us to transfer the knowledge we accumulate from one situation to another. They teach us to identify areas where we lack knowledge and how to access the help of those we trust to resolve the issue. Initially this support may be from parents, family or teachers but extends to include personal tutors or practice supervisors in clinical placements, whereas registered staff may turn to more experienced colleagues, unit leaders or members of other disciplines. The idea of life-wide learning, therefore, includes informal discussion, interest activities and learning within the family (Field, 2006). For example, we often discuss our views with others and, in the process, learn a different perspective on a problem from their response, or even some new knowledge they have shared with us. Being involved in an activity, such as sport, involves learning the rules of the game and new skills. Equally, incidental learning may occur during a formal preparation programme: for example, these could be skills such as typing or managing your time, or this learning could be more abstract; for example, developing professional attitudes such as care and compassion, as suggested by the 6 Cs. These skills and attitudes may not be taught formally but are aspects that you are likely to absorb as part of completing the nursing programme. In Case Study 2.1, Omar learned that it is acceptable for professionals to admit they do not know something and allow others to take the lead in providing the information. Equally importantly, Omar could identify a potential moment of learning and create a learning environment that was beneficial to him and, in doing this, create a learning environment for the group. As individuals, we should be able to define the different aspects of our lives that contribute to our learning. Consider Pippa's Case Study (2.2) as an example of informal learning taking place within her social group.

## Case Study 2.2: Pippa's difficult encounter

Pippa was in her final year of the mental health nursing programme. Pippa was married and had an 18-month-old daughter. Pippa's husband, Dave, was also a nurse who worked in the emergency department (ED). Ensuring patient confidentiality, Pippa spoke to Dave about a 15-year-old, named Jo who had been admitted after self-harming. Jo had been treated in the ED and transferred to the mental health setting where Pippa worked. After Pippa admitted Jo and completed the required documentation, Jo told Pippa that they had planned suicide but did not go through with it when confronted with the reality of the moment. Jo went on to say that their behaviour was triggered by realising that they identify as non-binary, that they were certain family would disown them due to religious beliefs, and Jo did not want their family to be informed. Pippa was upset by this episode and felt concerned as she had always taken for granted that parents would love and accept their children unconditionally. She had heard of an increasing number of young LGBTQ+ people leaving home due to non-acceptance, but this was the first time she had encountered a situation in real life.

Once home and talking to Dave about the situation, Pippa felt emotional as she could not imagine disowning her own daughter. She was not clear on what she found to be the biggest challenge – disowning one's own child or the fact that a young adult could be driven to such extreme behaviour through their assumptions of how their family would react to their sexuality.

During Pippa and Dave's discussion, Dave asked questions that helped Pippa to reflect more deeply on the situation. It became clear to Pippa that she had no idea how Jo's parents would react to this disclosure. In comparison, whilst her own parents were not staunchly religious, Pippa thought that they might have been influenced by what others (neighbours, family members, etc.) thought. Part of their hypothetical resistance could have been related to their lack of understanding of and exposure to LGBTQ+ people and culture and concerns about a difficult future for their daughter. By the end of the discussion Pippa came to understand that it was, perhaps too simplistic to consider religion only as being a barrier to acceptance. Pippa was embarrassed to realise that she had stereotyped Jo's parents and that she had already reached a conclusion without having met them or seen their interactions with Jo. Besides, she realised that she had taken it upon herself to 'save' Jo, rather than supporting and empowering them to resolve the situation with their parents.

Reading Case Study 2.2, you may relate to Pippa's response. You may see how Pippa's discussion with Dave contributed to her developing a more nuanced idea of Jo's family relationships. In Activity 2.1, you can now review your own life-wide learning.

### Activity 2.1 Critical thinking

For this activity, think about one thing you have learned since starting your nursing programme. Next, focus on everything about that thing you have learned outside of formal sessions, even though some may come from taught sessions or tutorials. Finally, develop a mind map of your learning that extends beyond classroom-based learning.

Suggested topics:

Active-listening, empathy, or time-management.

Watch the following to assist you https://www.youtube.com/watch?v=zVkF_EUShIo

You could use this app https://www.mindmaps.app/

*There is some guidance about this activity at the end of the chapter.*

Your map of learning will likely illustrate how extensive your learning is when considered outside the confines of the classroom and how this learning impacts your professional and personal life. Many students identify learning in areas such as assertiveness and communication that have benefited them as nurses but can also identify the impact this has on their personal lives. Examining your learning in this way helps to analyse its progression. We now consider the relationship to life-long learning.

# What is life-long learning?

Banks et al. (2007) suggest that life-long learning extends from childhood into old age and includes how we manage interpersonal interactions and our beliefs, and how we deal with new experiences. As you can imagine, we are often not aware of this learning. Similarly, Jarvis (2024) considers life-long learning as a process of learning that continues across our lives. Nursing practice requires continuing professional development (CPD), the life-long process of learning that develops and maintains competences, enhances professional practice and growth in an ever-evolving climate of change (Hakvoort et al., 2022). The Nursing and Midwifery Council (NMC) Code (NMC, 2018b) advocates that nurses continue to learn to maintain the currency of their knowledge, but also to have an enquiring attitude to their practice and performance. For example, the section *Practise effectively* (items 6.1 and 6.2) which is part of *Platform 1: Being an accountable professional* of the NMC's *Future Nurse: Standards of Proficiency for Registered Nurses* (NMC, 2018a), as presented in Scenario 2.1, relates to communication, commitment and competence – three of the 6 Cs. These require you to be open to new experiences while recognising limitations to your knowledge and taking the necessary action to resolve the limitation. Without which, we are unable to provide true holistic person-centred care (Jackson, 2025). Thus, life-long learning comes with an individual responsibility actively to pursue learning in addition to your preparation programme. Life-long learning differs from life-long education in that 'learning' is about developing your understanding across the spectrum of your life, whereas 'education' may refer to ideas that are taught (Jarvis, 2024).

# What is life-deep learning?

Moon (2000) explains how reflection on new situations takes place within the context of what we already know; we reflect on new experiences by viewing them through the lens of our life as we have known it and what is familiar. Life-long learning in a life-wide sense invites an approach to learning that includes how others have influenced you, you could say that life-long and life-wide learning takes place within the context of life-deep learning. Banks et al. (2007) indicate that life-deep learning includes moral, ethical, spiritual, and social values that guide what we believe, how we act and how we view ourselves and others. These authors suggest that we construct our lives around symbols, and family life is instrumental in our learning as it teaches us to understand symbols of communication providing us with a multitude of skills and tasks. The learning available to family members does, however, take place according to our specific family **culture** and tradition. We can understand the powerful nature of this learning when we are confronted with other cultural beliefs and habits. We will come back to an idea called *cultural competency* later in this book. You can see how life-long aspects of learning relate to who you are within your relationships, which is linked to the culture you have grown up in, your history, hopes and ideas and your goals. For example, how does your experience of learning in its widest sense influence your approaches to ongoing learning? This might relate to the way feelings produced by past learning experiences are taken forward and how they influence your engagement with further learning. An example could be the 'mental block' some students have with numeracy assessments, which is often related to their earlier school experience.

Challenges of learning to understand communication symbols can be seen in how we sometimes struggle to interpret verbal and non-verbal communication and are why virtual communications such as email and social media can be misunderstood. We learn language and behavioural symbols in relation to roles such as child, parent, pupil, or student, and these are possibly very different from that of a healthcare professional. You may already have noticed that there are different expectations of you, as a student nurse, to previous expectations.

## Activity 2.2 Looking for symbols

Please take a few minutes to think of any different expectations regarding your language or behaviour that you may have noticed since starting the nursing programme. To apply this activity, consider a minority or marginalised group that you might be unfamiliar with. Often by reflecting on vulnerable and marginalised groups that are unfamiliar, we can critically reflect on our norms and values, gain insight into our levels of acceptance and identify how we view people in terms of their being unique individuals and from a holistic perspective. Write these down and then cluster them according to whether you think the language or behaviour symbol is a professional expectation or whether they are peer expectations due to you being in a new group.

*As this activity is based on your own experiences, there is no outline answer at the end of the chapter.*

Looking back at what we have covered, it is clear that we are complex individuals whose learning is influenced by multiple factors. Although healthcare draws on knowledge relating to the body, there are many areas where we need to stay abreast of developments. Think back to the concerns raised in Chapter 1 about how the body is viewed, and to the outcome skills at the start of this chapter relating to healthcare organisation and structure. As healthcare becomes more complex and more impersonal, healthcare staff members need to take a more holistic view that considers emotional and social dimensions when working with people across the spectrum of humanity (Howatson-Jones & Thurgate, 2014). Learning involves social elements through our interactions, emotional aspects perceived by how we feel about things and cognitive parts representing our thinking (Illeris, 2009). These all influence our sense of self and our learning. Life-long learning encompasses several dimensions that interconnect according to your intentions and opportunities (Figure 2.1).

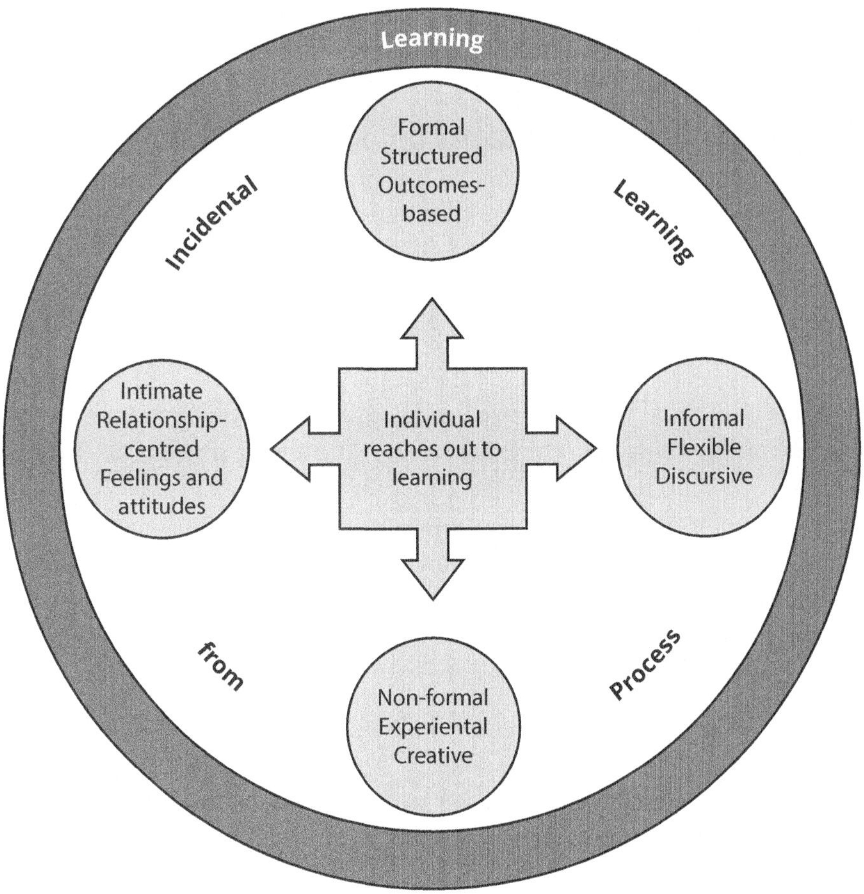


*Figure 2.1* Some dimensions of learning

As suggested in Figure 2.1, formal learning is usually directed towards a learning outcome. For example, the nursing programme is based on a curriculum, approved by the regulatory body, covering what you need to know to work as a registered nurse. The outcome by the end of the programme is the ability to function at a specific level as a registered nurse. Incidental learning occurs alongside formal learning activities and is influenced by the quality of these activities and experiences. Informal (life-wide) learning relates to the discussions with your peers and patients, which help to develop your thinking and knowledge. Experiential (life-long) learning relates to what you learn from dealing with different situations. Relationship-centred (life-deep) learning is about how you learn to manage attitudes and feelings within your encounters with others.

As individuals, we are at the centre of our learning. It is up to us whether we engage with it and are aware of what we have learned. How we integrate different ways of learning is another form of learning and a major part of life-long learning. To do this, we need to reflect on our learning, build on what we already know, make connections between different forms of learning, and consider our development. Consider the case study below involving Francine's integration of her learning to identify how integrated reflection might contribute to further learning.

## Case Study 2.3: Francine's integration of her learning

Francine was an overseas student, from Cameroon, where she was the middle child of five siblings. As both her parents worked, she had often helped with her siblings and consequently learned the skills of looking after herself at the same time. To her, a nursing qualification was important to enable her to support herself and contribute to the family.

Francine was in the first year of her learning disability nursing programme and was learning about the human body, person-centred nursing practice and her developing professional identity. She enjoyed the practical aspects of the course because she could connect some of what she was learning to her previous knowledge of caring for her siblings in terms of hygiene and bathing, feeding and elimination. Francine did find some of the theoretical elements hard to grasp, especially the clinical science sessions, which seemed to use terminology she did not understand. Francine reflected on what she could do.

On reflection, Francine recognised that she was learning a new scientific language. At home in Cameroon everyone spoke in French and some English, and she remembered how she had found it easier to learn English from her friends. Maybe she could draw on her bilingual experiences to help her learn this scientific terminology. Francine decided this would be easier if she could share this with others and so asked some of her class if they wanted to form a revision group. The students in the study group were from all four fields of nursing (adult, child, learning disability and mental health) and agreed to meet, informally, weekly for 2 hours to go over what they had learned in the previous session and fill in the gaps. Some of the revision group had other learning needs and one student, Michael, volunteered to summarise their learning into an ongoing revision document for them all to use.

Michael checked the accuracy of the document with the module tutor who was impressed by the group's initiative.

Francine was surprised and pleased at her success in arranging this group. When she reflected on this, she recognised that some of her experiences of managing herself were also instrumental in the organisation and design of her learning and developing assertiveness. By drawing together different threads of her learning she was also able to contribute to her further learning.

Having read this Case Study, you may have started to reflect on your own life-long learning and how different aspects might connect to make something new. Try to relate this exercise back to Activity 2.2 and analyse what this might mean for you. Activity 2.3 offers you an opportunity to think about your life-long learning and reach some conclusions.

## Activity 2.3 Reflection

Think about your learning since you started your nursing programme. If you are in your first year of the programme, you may want to consider the following questions:

- How has my view of nursing changed and why?
- What skills have I learnt?
- How has my identity changed?
- How have my values changed?

If you are further on in the programme you may want to think about the following:

- What areas of my knowledge have changed and why?
- What areas of my knowledge do I need to develop further and why?

If you are an experienced practitioner, you may want to think about the following:

- What changes have happened in healthcare since I started in my practitioner role?
- What knowledge change has this required from me?
- How did I develop this knowledge?
- How have I developed my evidence base?
- What further goals do I have for my learning?

*There is some guidance about this activity at the end of the chapter.*

When completing this activity, please consider different contexts and ways in which you increase your knowledge and evidence base over time. We now look at some contexts where learning takes place.

# Contexts in which learning takes place

The theoretical learning that you undertake provides you with essential background information to inform your practice. Similarly, practice helps you make sense of the theory you have learnt but can also inform theory when something new is identified; for example, the way a patient responds to the nursing interventions you provide. Your placements are a context for learning from the experiences you have there. People are all different, as are the circumstances in which they are nursed. Each of these experiences offers an opportunity for learning. So, with many scenarios contained within each clinical shift, one could argue that it is not possible, as some students state, not to be able to learn anything in a particular placement area. It is so important to be aware of the learning opportunities that arise and be proactive in using them to your advantage.

Learning, whether undertaken in university or in practice, can also be shared with others. Learning as a group is a valuable way of turning ideas into articulated thinking, as was illustrated in Francine's Case Study. The process of explaining something to someone else shows us what we really understand about an issue and, at the same time, the feedback from others opens the possibilities of further thinking to develop understanding. The virtual world provides another avenue for expanding our ideas and learning when others are not immediately available to share ideas with.

The virtual nursing world can be both a public and a private space for learning; for example, virtual learning environment discussion boards may be viewed by many course participants and are public. Contributions may, correspondingly, be less spontaneous and more considered before being placed in such a public domain, because of possible concerns about feeling exposed to criticism (Price, 2024b, p. 102; Thompson & Thompson, 2023, p. 93). In this context it is sometimes harder to acknowledge unfinished thinking. Nevertheless, electronic resources can provide opportunities for learning that are individually focused. For example, you can look up the action of a particular drug or disease process or identify the latest research underpinning a particular nursing intervention. This learning can be accessed and completed in private and at your own pace.

There may be times when you are too shy to ask and may be tempted to rely solely on virtual sources for information that do not expose you to the scrutiny of others, but do not underestimate the importance of testing your ideas with peers and educators. Only through doing this can you establish whether you are thinking along the correct lines. However, it is important to remember that not all electronic sources or sites are credible, and some information may be biased. Make sure that such learning is related to some framework for learning to help you stay focused. You will also need to have access to reliable guidance to help evaluate what you have found and avoid mistakes. An example may be looking something up and then discussing this further with your practice supervisor or course tutor. In the case study about Francine above, the revision guide created by the group was checked with the module tutor by Michael, for accuracy.

This not only helps to avoid mistakes but may also help to share learning that is beneficial with others.

When trying anything for the first time there is an element of learning from the mistakes you make. Mistakes can be a valuable way of learning when you reflect on what went wrong, analyse the processes that led to the mistake and consider what you can do to avoid making the same mistake again. Taking responsibility for what went wrong enables new ideas to develop (Rogers & Freiberg, 1994; Thompson & Thompson, 2023, p. 75). Mistakes, although unpleasant in their possible consequences and challenges to self-confidence, also provide emotional learning about how to manage anxiety and disappointment. And how to seek resolution in a positive way (Barchard, 2022). Support for such learning may come from family members or close peers, or through the encouragement of colleagues. Nevertheless, it requires time and motivation to reflect on what has been learned. To help you understand some of these points relating to learning from mistakes, please consider Case Study 2.4 and then complete Activity 2.4.

## Case Study 2.4: Kevin's mistake

Kevin was working with residents diagnosed with cognitive impairment on the secure unit in a residential home and was in the first year of his mental health nursing programme. He had been working in the home for two weeks and was starting to get to know the people and processes. Today Kevin was looking after Jim, who had a diagnosis of Korsakoffs syndrome. Jim had had a urinary accident in his carpeted room and Kevin went to inform his practice supervisor, Briony, to find out what to do, assuming that this would be dealt with differently to what he would do at home. Briony told Kevin he would need to use a spillage kit to remove the urine from the carpet and she would join him shortly but first needed to finish giving her residents their drugs.

Kevin found the spillage kit and wanted to appear helpful and show initiative as Jim was attempting to clear the spillage himself. Besides, the instructions appeared straightforward, so he proceeded to use the kit before Briony joined him. On entering the room Briony found Kevin coughing with his eyes streaming. She immediately helped him to wash his eyes out and told him to go off duty and go to the Emergency Department (ED) for a check-up. Instead, Kevin sat in the staff room downstairs for half an hour until Briony went off duty and, as he felt better, he went back upstairs to complete his hours.

The next day Briony asked Kevin what the ED staff had said. He replied that he had not gone to the ED. Briony was upset about this but remained professional. When she and Kevin had completed their work, she asked Kevin to come into the seminar room with her to discuss the episode and complete an incident report.

### Activity 2.4 Reflection

- What are the significant aspects of this scenario and why?
- What questions might Briony have for Kevin?
- Why is it important for Kevin to reflect on the actions/inactions that he undertook?
- Which of the 6 Cs are relevant in the scenario and why?

If you are a student, you might want to reflect on a situation where perhaps you tried to resolve a situation that did not go entirely to plan. If you are an experienced practitioner, think about what you want to consider as the practice supervisor.

*There are outline answers to these questions at the end of the chapter.*

Case study 2.4 may have identified difficulties involved when trying to fit into a new environment and team. It may also have highlighted some problems that could arise from inaction. Both are contexts of learning, and we need to be able to link the formal and the less formal. Please consider the features of formal and less formal ways of learning below.

# Features of learning in formal and less formal ways

Features of formal learning involve codifying information into our thinking. What this means is that the information is often already offered in the form of categories and theories, which we embed in our thinking according to specific set outcomes. This may make concepts easier to grasp but could also inhibit the development of different interpretations and restrict lateral thinking. Thompson and Thompson (2023) tell us that reflecting on formal learning can help to negate such effects by discovering alternative views. Consider some features in your formal learning by completing Activity 2.5.

### Activity 2.5 Critical thinking

Think about a recent class you attended as part of your programme. What features of learning can you identify by considering the following questions?

- How did the lesson start?
- What were you asked to do during the lesson?
- How did the lesson finish?
- What did you learn?
- Did you do anything further to aid your learning after the lesson and, if so, what did you do?

If you are an experienced practitioner, consider a recent CPD session.

*There is an outline answer to this activity at the end of the chapter.*

Formal learning provides initial knowledge for practice and is often the start of professional learning. However, sharing experiences with peers in a less formal way is an important feature of professional learning. Through sharing experiences informally, different interpretations, based on subjective experiences, are offered and explored, allowing debate and reconsideration of the conclusions that might be reached. The feature of this learning is its evolving and discursive nature, which means that it is flexible and responsive, but therefore it can be difficult to quantify this form of evidence. Personal learning can help support professional practice and is another feature of less formal ways of learning through reworking personal knowledge within the professional setting. An example might be having the ability to speak another language and using this to translate in the professional setting. Integration of personal and professional learning supports a holistic approach to health and social care. Next, consider some features of your less formal learning by completing Activity 2.6.

### Activity 2.6 Critical thinking

Think about a recent discussion you had in practice. What features of learning can you identify by examining the following?

- What prompted the discussion?
- What were the key arguments made?
- What was the outcome of the discussion?
- What did you learn?
- Did you do anything further to aid your learning?

*There is an outline answer to this activity at the end of the chapter.*

Within Activity 2.5 and Activity 2.6 you will have had an opportunity to compare different forms of learning. We will now look at types of knowledge and ways of knowing that are relevant to the healthcare practitioner.

# Types of knowledge and ways of knowing

Theories and protocols are important for identifying what knowledge is expected of the professional learner. Examples include theories of communication and psychological processing, how the human body works, disease effects, infection control and much more. Protocols, such as National Institute for Health and Care Excellence (NICE) guidelines, relate to identification of what is required within a particular situation such as assessment procedures, what to do when someone experiences a stroke or cardiac arrest, or how to prepare somebody for an operation. These constitute professional knowledge and should reflect evidence-based and best-practice standards. In other words, these would be professional ways of knowing that relate to the meaning that a professional derives from a situation through experience and from applying theory and evidence to practice. Additionally, practical knowledge relates to knowing how to do things and developing the skills required to carry them out.

## Aesthetic knowing

Personal knowledge comes from the *life-world* of individuals (Jarvis, 2006) in that it comes from their background, culture, with whom they interact and the activities in which they are involved. It also relates to how individuals see themselves and others. Personal knowledge develops from reflecting on events and making sense of situations and is illustrated in Figure 2.1 as 'Incidental Learning from Process'. Over time, layers of experience may filter into the unconscious and re-emerge later as intuitive knowing. The following short case study is offered as an example of how the different types of knowledge and knowing may all interlink in your practice of healthcare.

### Case Study 2.5: Suzy's day

Suzy was a final year children's nursing apprentice and was working in an **oncology** setting, which she enjoyed. There were clear guidelines for when patients were due to have particular treatments, and Suzy had spent today discussing some of these with her practice supervisor, Ben, to gain a better understanding. Ben had first explored Suzy's knowledge of the relevant clinical science relating to various types of cancers, in particular the cell development cycle and how this was important to determine treatment phases.

The discussion between Suzy and Ben then moved forward to her assessment, which was due soon. Suzy identified that many of the patients required regular blood tests and, although Suzy had been trained in **venepuncture** in her previous role as a healthcare assistant (HCA), she understood that she was not allowed to undertake this in her current role as an apprentice because of differences in responsibility and accountability. Suzy was also able to articulate the differences in undertaking venepuncture on an adult when compared to a child. Ben highlighted, however, that Suzy was always ready with the required equipment when colleagues needed to take a sample, which they valued. She had also been quick to identify **phlebitis** in a patient, which was undoubtedly due to her previous experience.

Ben asked Suzy to reflect on why she enjoyed working in this particular setting and what she had learned. When thinking about this, Suzy identified that dignity, respect and compassion were important values for her. Supporting children with cancer, and their parents, was fulfilling because of the opportunity to really listen and attend to someone else's situation, as she was not able to be involved in some of the treatments. From this she had learned what therapeutic relationship and communication actually mean in practice and they were no longer just an abstract idea. Suzy told Ben that reflection on this placement had enabled her to bring the abstract idea of the 6 Cs to life through the identification of her values and the depth of communication she had practised. She felt, because she had 'lived' this learning, it would stay with her.

Through reading the Case Study you may have noted how professional, practical and personal knowledge are integrated in a typical day. The role of reflection in achieving this is paramount, so we end this chapter by highlighting how learning is related to reflection.

# Learning and reflection

Processes of learning carry mixed emotions which can hinder learning experiences due to feelings of anxiety or uncertainty. It is worth remembering that learning reams of facts does not embed understanding or application of learning. To transform learning into something that you can apply in different situations with different people and at different times, we need to reflect on learning to enable examination of what has actually been learned. It is through reflection that connections can be made for:

- life-wide and life-long learning;
- learning and life-deep learning;
- different types of learning;
- different types of knowledge and knowing;
- the evidence base being used;
- how to manage emotions;
- what values and beliefs are developing;
- what alternatives are available;
- what the likely outcomes are;
- what nursing is.

## Chapter summary

This chapter examines some of the issues listed above and offers a range of opportunities to make some of these connections through the case studies, activities and scenarios provided. Undertaking the activities allows you to apply some of the ideas around life-wide, life-long and life-deep learning in different settings and at different stages of the nurse preparation programme. This is a crucial part of continuing life-long learning as set out in the NMC's *Future Nurse: Standards of Proficiency for Registered Nurses* (NMC, 2018a) at the start of the chapter, to meet the challenges of healthcare evolving and changing. How to explore life-wide learning in greater depth is the subject of Chapter 3.

## Brief outline answers

In this section, answers to the chapter's activities will be outlined and explained.

## Activity 2.1 Critical thinking

Your answer might have included:

- how to communicate in different groups;
- how to communicate with different people or in different situations;
- developing friendships;
- using the internet to find information, writing up notes, reading;
- learning to drive, swim, play a sport;
- learning to cook, manage finance, become a parent;
- learning to problem solve.

As indicated when the activity was introduced, you might find it helpful to develop a visual map of all your learning first and then group various categories together.

## Activity 2.3 Reflection

If you are a novice practitioner in your first year, your answer may have considered:

- Nursing is hard work and emotionally challenging.
- Skills learnt in the first year include recording nursing observations such as temperature, pulse, respiration and blood pressure and oxygen saturations, and undertaking urinalysis, bed bathing and basic wound care, administering injections, checking medications with the practice supervisor and caring for urinary catheters.
- Identity changes may include becoming more assertive and confident.

If you are further on in your nurse preparation programme, you may have thought about:

- having more knowledge about how clinical science applies in practice;
- a need to develop wider knowledge of pharmacology and pathophysiology to understand treatment options.

If you are an experienced practitioner, you may have thought about:

- increasing use of technology in nursing observations and interventions;
- the move to an all-graduate profession for nursing;
- returning to further formal academic study;
- investigating new opportunities and knowledge requirements in nursing.

## Activity 2.4 Reflection

In Case Study 2.2, Kevin did not follow his practice supervisor's instructions, and tried to do things on his own before he was been given the relevant information. When you are new to any environment it is important to be oriented to the correct processes and procedures, and view supervision as support rather than a sign of weakness. By not following his practice supervisor's instructions, Kevin's actions resulted in poor infection control and personal safety risks. The questions Briony might have discussed with Kevin in the seminar room could have included why he did not wait for her before starting to use the spillage kit and why he did not get himself checked in the ED. Briony could then use Kevin's answers as teaching aids to demonstrate how using her support could provide more positive outcomes. Briony might ask Kevin to write a reflection about this for her and his personal tutor to consolidate his learning from this.

Kevin's initiative is commendable, but understanding potential risks is vital. Care, communication, and commitment may have been three of the 6 Cs motivating Kevin to undertake the action he did. He wanted to care for Jim and his living environment and was committed to his role of a nurse, not wanting to burden Briony unduly, and that he was not above doing 'menial' tasks. Communication is key – the written instructions on the spillage kit appeared straightforward, but did not give adequate warning of potential dangers. Briony assumed that Kevin would implicitly understand that she was not suggesting he wait because of the seeming 'simplicity' of the task at hand, but rather because it was a more complex and risk-laden procedure. This could be a point of reflection for Briony, namely, to reflect on how she communicates a potentially hazardous activity.

As part of this exercise, it is recommended that you consult the NMC Code (2018b). Kevin's actions placed Briony in a difficult position, potentially breaching NMC Code areas, such as *practising effectively* (item 7.4), which states that a nurse should check people's understanding to minimise misunderstanding and mistakes. Similarly, Kevin may have put the resident, Jim, at risk from the fumes, which could have breached item 8.5. Risk assessment is essential for both service users and staff, with significant consequences if not followed.

As a student you may want to reflect on:

- how you set boundaries and how you assess the risk of what you do;
- what makes you want to try things for yourself, e.g. not wanting to make demands on your practice supervisor, you feel restricted in your development by not being able to make decisions yourself, or you are aware of your learning style;
- how clear you have been in discussing your plans for the placement – in other words, have you been proactive in setting your learning outcomes, have you discussed your learning style with your practice supervisor and which style of support works for you, etc.?
- if you find you are unable to approach your practice supervisor openly, why is this and what action can you take to improve the relationship?

As an experienced practitioner thinking as a practice supervisor, you might consider:

- how to maintain a supportive learning relationship while correcting practice;
- how to construct feedback to support safe and effective practice;
- the need to involve university representatives;
- how to act on the learning results.

## Activity 2.5 Critical thinking

Your answer may have identified that the lesson started with the learning objectives of what you were expected to learn. You may have been asked to discuss some of the concepts in smaller groups and apply these to practice scenarios. The lesson may have finished by summarising the main points. You may have identified that you remembered some of the key points and may have undertaken some further reading of your notes. You could also have undertaken self-study to clarify terminology or concepts you did not fully understand, or you may have created a glossary of terms to which you can refer.

As an experienced practitioner thinking about a CPD session, you may have considered how the lesson started by enquiring about your present knowledge of the topic. During the session you are likely to have discussed application to your practice, in small groups. The session could have finished with a summary of the key points and guidance on directed study. You may have tried to fit in the directed study around your workload and expanded your learning through further discussion with colleagues. You could have used the insights and knowledge gained from the session to consider critically the strengths and weaknesses in your area of work.

## Activity 2.6 Critical thinking

Your answer could have identified that a patient issue stimulated the discussion. Key points of this discussion are likely to have included background information about the issue, who should be involved and possible solutions. The outcome is likely to have been an agreement on the solution to be implemented. Perhaps you thought about the intervention and considered whether alternatives may have been more appropriate. You could also have wondered on what evidence the decision for the intervention was based. You may have identified learning about decision-making, team working and problem-solving. You may have reflected on this further afterwards. Have you noticed that it seems more natural to reflect on situations that are based on relationships?

The aspects of learning and reflection identified in this activity will possibly seem quite logical and obvious. Hopefully, they are, but the objective of this is to help you become aware of the importance of these activities and to remind you that this seemingly obvious activity is part of professional practice and is included in the NMC's Code (2018b).

## Further reading

**Price, B.** (2024). *Critical thinking and writing in nursing* (6th ed.). Sage.

This book assists students in developing critical thinking and reflection. It explains what critical thinking is and its importance within nursing practice, how to use these skills in practical contexts and how readers can demonstrate their abilities in written form.

**Qalehsari, M. Q. et al.** (2017). Lifelong learning strategies in nursing: A systematic review. *Electron Physician,* Oct. *9*(10), 5541–5550. www.ncbi.nlm.nih.gov/pmc/articles/PMC5718860/

This article identifies the benefits of facilitating life-long learning attributes in nurse education programmes to enhance care.

**Thomas, C.** (2023). Sources of knowledge for evidence-based care. In P. Ellis (Ed.), *Evidence-based practice in nursing* (5th ed.). Sage.

This is a clear and concise guide on how to search for and access relevant evidence via electronic information sources and digital media.

## Useful websites

**https://helpfulprofessor.com/lifelong-learning/**

A useful blog post containing tips for life-long learning.

**https://www.legislation.gov.uk/**

Most (but not all) types of legislation and their accompanying explanatory documents.

**https://www.nice.org.uk/guidance/HTE21**

**https://www.nice.org.uk/guidance/ng131/chapter/recommendations**

Robotic surgery guidance resources and information.

**https://learning.nspcc.org.uk/child-protection-system/gillick-competence-fraser-guidelines**

Information on capacity and decision making for children when considering their wishes and keeping them safe.

**https://youtu.be/_PUxv3BAFM8?si=V56nXQNZHTqBGJJj**

A very inclusive YouTube video showing how to mind map effectively.

# Chapter 3 Autobiographical reflection and learning

## NMC Future Nurse: Standards of Proficiency for Registered Nurses

This chapter will address the following platforms and proficiencies:

**Platform 1: Being an accountable professional**

1.5 Understand the demands of professional practice and demonstrate how to recognise signs of vulnerability in themselves or their colleagues and the action required to minimise risks to health.

1.10 Demonstrate resilience and emotional intelligence and be capable of explaining the rationale that influences their judgements and decisions in routine, complex and challenging situations.

1.17 Take responsibility for continuous self-reflection, seeking and responding to support and feedback to develop their professional knowledge and skills.

## Chapter aims

After reading this chapter you will be able to:

- consider how reflection integrates the personal with the professional, drawing on experiences from all areas of life;
- complete a life story construction exercise;
- creatively explore your experiences by reflecting on your life story and **life world**;
- integrate reflection and learning with a sense of developing values and a developing identity;
- reflect on aspects of your life that may also reveal societal issues.

### Case Study 3.1: Amina's autobiographical experience

Amina is a student nurse; she has a 12-year-old brother and an 8-year-old sister. Amina's parents work shifts; she often looks after her siblings.

One evening, she noticed that her sister Astur looked tired and was becoming distressed with the noise from the television. She suggested that Astur go to bed, but when she went to say goodnight, she noticed that Astur looked very ashen. Amina remembered a campaign for the warning signs of meningitis she had recently seen on social media. She recalled that Astur had been avoiding the lights and noises of the television, and she was pale. Their mother had recently explained that a rash can be harder to see on dark skin so she checked the paler areas of Astur's body (the palms of her hands, soles of her feet, roof of her mouth and her abdomen). She took a glass and rolled it over the spots that were visible in these areas, and they did not fade.

Amina immediately called their mother and an ambulance. It was confirmed that Astur did have meningitis and that her vigilance ensured Astur received treatment early. Amina was commended by both her mother and the healthcare team. She was proud of her actions and relieved that Astur recovered, although she did wonder whether she could have recognised the symptoms sooner.

This episode helped her when deciding to become a children's nurse and was writing her statement to apply for entry to the programme. She was able to reflect and identify some strengths. She concluded that she possessed the observational and decision-making skills required of a nurse and understood there were emotional consequences to the caring profession.

As a student nurse, Amina reflected on how emotional residue from caring work may be different when managing situations personally or professionally. She used her autobiographical experience to develop discussion with her peers about the observation of symptoms and disease as well as the emotional consequences of critical incidents. In doing this, Amina used her personal, ethnic and cultural history to help peers identify the possible differences in symptom presentation between fair and dark-skinned patients. Through sharing this story, Amina reached an understanding of herself as being a capable and caring person, able to cope in an unexpected situation. She also realised that she would benefit from support to manage her emotions constructively and use them in her thinking and decision-making.

# Introduction

This chapter started with an example scenario to illustrate how your life story helps you make sense of your capabilities and progress as a student nurse. You entered the nursing programme with a variety of experiences, and these influence your perception and experience of yourself, of others and of practice. In Case Study 3.1, Amina's capabilities are affirmed, but through further reflection she identified areas she could develop further. Developing reflective insight is an important starting point for any person entering a caring profession, and particularly nursing. Such insight explains why we react and think in certain ways, what resources in the form of family and friends and personal knowledge are available to us and what the possibilities may be for development and change.

When talking about life stories we are referring to our autobiographies. In other words, how do our family, school, work and social experiences and formal learning make us who we are, and influence how we think and react, our norms and values and our ambitions? Reflecting on these areas of our lives can sometimes be challenging, painful or confrontational, as well as enriching and exciting. To do this effectively, you need courage and commitment – two of the 6 Cs. The point here is that we cannot separate our personal and professional entities – the two are inextricably linked and any change in one will result in a change in the other. Looking at Amina's example in Case Study 3.1, we can see that the unresolved emotional issues she carried from the experience with her younger sister has made her more aware of emotional risks associated with caring for children. This insight into her own response seems to motivate her to care for peers and colleagues by alerting them of potential issues. Had she not had this personal experience, it is possible that she would have been unaware of potential emotional risks to her and her colleagues. It could be said that Amina may become more extreme in her perception of emotional risk and become overburdened through an inability to filter her experiences. Additionally, Amina could feel responsible for 'protecting' her peers and colleagues; this is an aspect that needs further consideration and will be discussed in more depth in Chapter 9.

This chapter introduces the idea of **autobiographical** reflection to advance nursing knowledge in different ways. Firstly, by defining autobiographical reflection before considering how to integrate personal and professional experience, and the importance of doing so. Next, you are invited to construct your own autobiography with guidance on the key points for inclusion. Then this is followed by further guidance on how to examine and reflect on your autobiography. The chapter ends by looking at how societal issues may be given meaning through subjective experience.

## What is autobiographical reflection?

As people progress through life, they begin to develop a life history. This history, just like any other, charts the timeline of events and changes that have come about. It also includes motives for actions, how situations have been shaped, how the individual has been shaped by events and their aspirations for the future. From the experiences that individuals have in their lives, personal knowledge develops. Experiences will be diverse because they result from the ways in which we encounter the world and make sense of it through interacting with others (Boud & Miller, 2002). This resonates with Bhabha's (2012) work which describes a 'third space'. This arises from one individual connecting with another or a group and, through shared experiences and perceptions, creating a hybrid way of perceiving the world. For example, starting a nursing programme exposes us to many different people and types of learning. Others, such as practice supervisors, colleagues, lecturers and peers, respond to our efforts to interact and understand; we internalise the feedback they provide as knowledge of personal ability. Read Case Study 3.2 about Callum's biographical account of school to identify what learning he might have taken forward from this experience.

## Case Study 3.2: Callum's biographical account of school

Callum had struggled with learning at primary school and was dyslexic. He was often made fun of by his peers. However, he excelled at sport, particularly rugby, where he demonstrated good leadership qualities as team captain. The nature of the game meant that players got injured and Callum would assist because he had taken a first-aid course; he enjoyed the course because of its practical content, which he found easy to understand. After leaving school Callum went into nursing because of the practical nature of the work and before it required university-based study.

After qualifying as a nurse Callum completed mainly clinically practical courses relating to his nursing work. He progressed some way in his career but realised that to progress further he would need to complete formal study, because nursing education, including continuing professional development, was now located within universities. Callum worked with the **Specific Learning Differences** (SpLD) team from the university to help him write a reflective account of the learning he had achieved over the years, to submit in a portfolio of evidence. This attracted academic credits equivalent to a diploma.

Callum enjoyed undertaking this reflective work as it suited his learning style. The SpLD team offered continual feedback so that his final portfolio was presentable and relatively error-free. Callum achieved a grade of 55 per cent and felt encouraged to continue with the degree.

## Activity 3.1 Reflection

- What learning is Callum taking forward from school?
- What learning is Callum taking forward from his portfolio study experience?

*There is an outline answer to this activity at the end of the chapter.*

Case Study 3.2 identifies that experiences of learning can be both positive and challenging. Horsdal (2012, p. 25) suggests that the way we use our senses and communicate affects the development of our 'social brain'. Sharing our experiences with empathetic listeners, such as Callum did with the SpLD team means that we can retrace our steps in a supported way and consequently learn from our experiences. In such a way experiences can be transformed through autobiographical reflection. An autobiography turns these experiences into an account of what has been lived through and the meaning that has been attached to this as part of a personal history. Autobiography reviews individual experiences within the life history and reflection scrutinises links between them to explore how the past might be influencing the present. In doing so, we find creative ways to address situations and problems by drawing on personal knowledge that has come from personal history. In this way, autobiographical reflection helps to make sense of past experiences within an individual life history and what is being taken forward, raising the possibility of change. This is also the case for professional experiences, certainly at the start of your professional career. The only reference upon which to reflect is our personal experience. As we build our professional experience, so we have more 'professional landmarks' to reflect on and, in time, we may feel that our 'professional values' differ from our 'personal values'. This is an interesting phenomenon which is why continual reflection on, and awareness of, how we are developing is so important. Not doing this can lead to alienation from yourself and those close to you. Just think for a moment of the things you experience in your first placement of your nursing programme; often you see and experience more challenging and emotional situations than some people experience in their entire lives. Buckley et al. (2024a) remind us how reflection on your experiences – good and bad – helps to develop resilience and manage more effectively with things that cross both professional and personal paths.

We do not always pay attention to the experiences that we encounter and therefore may not recognise their value in terms of what has been learned or what can be translated to different circumstances and situations. Equally, there may be times when it feels like we have reached an impasse by becoming too overwhelmed by the situation to be able to move forward. For example, learning anatomy and physiology can be difficult for some people and yet these are integral parts of nursing knowledge. If you have artistic attributes, these could potentially play a part in how you perceive things and respond to them. You may be more comfortable with the art of nursing than the science. Acknowledging this is a first step to dealing with potential difficulties that may arise in learning the language and structure of scientific theories. This is known as "finding the self" which can be accessed by unlocking life experiences such as resilience and motivation (McClunie-Trust et al., 2025).

Autobiographical reflection is not limited to clinical or negative experiences; we learn that we can learn from all experiences. It is a way of making sense of what is happening, set within the context of our lives. By focusing attention on our life history, we can identify how we can renegotiate a position and deal with the challenge we are facing (Horsdal, 2007). This renegotiation is called **agency,** and, by this, we can take control of our lives. We use our life resources to construct strategies for developing and managing change (McClunie-Trust et al., 2024). Therefore, in the example of the artistic student nurse, it might be that creating revision notes using colour and drawing is one way to surmount an obstacle to understanding scientific concepts. Although there have been numerous definitions and descriptions of reflection, in essence they can be related back to work by Boud et al. (1985, p. 19), indicating that reflection, in the first instance, requires:

- returning to experience;
- attending to feelings;
- re-evaluating experience;
- planning change.

This is not dissimilar to the reflective cycle suggested by Barksby et al. (2015, p. 22). In this model, the authors recommend seven stages in the reflective cycle which clearly mirror Boud et al. (1985):

- R: *Recall* (the events).
- E: *Examine* (your responses).
- F: (Acknowledge) *feelings*.
- L: *Learn* (from the experience).
- E: *Explore*(options).
- C: *Create* (a plan of action).
- T: (Set) timescale.

## Activity 3.2 Reflection

Look back at Case study 3.2 (Callum's biographical account of school and learning as a nurse) and consider the following.

- What meaning do you think he has attached to his experiences?
- What creative ways might he find to help his learning?

*There is an outline answer to this activity at the end of the chapter.*

Autobiographical reflection explores personal learning in how the past is combined with perceptions of sensations within the present (Jarvis, 2024). Such reflection involves thinking about how, in the first instance, to construct the autobiographical account in terms of what to include, what seems relevant in the present moment and why. For example, it can be helpful to gather autobiographical experiences of learning – what Dominice (2000) calls *writing an educational biography* – to develop an understanding of personal learning processes by reflecting on diverse learning experiences through the life history. Such autobiographical reflection looks at learning in its widest sense of formal and informal experience. This can be a valuable exercise in terms of both academic and practice learning. It can be challenging when you do not receive the grade you had anticipated for an assignment, or you are given points to improve on by your practice supervisor. It is worth reflecting on how you receive this information: do you accept it graciously, possibly asking for further clarification? Or do you become defensive, feel embarrassed or feel that you are a failure? Or do you blame your tutor? These are exactly the valuable points to reflect on – why do you feel this way? Is it your 'voice' or is it the 'voice' of a teacher at secondary school? Is what the teacher then said still valid? You are, after all, older, have more life experience and are in a vastly different situation. This is a strong reflective topic; often nursing students become paralysed at the thought of numeracy, research or science-related subjects when, on further exploration, one finds that they have had a challenging or traumatic experience in school – perhaps failing an exam or feeling humiliated in front of their peers. It is helpful to understand why you think or are afraid that this will happen again and, possibly more importantly, why you think that your reaction will be the same. These are all excellent topics for reflection.

Apply consideration of autobiographical experience to your own life by completing Activity 3.3.

### Activity 3.3 Critical thinking

Spend a little time thinking of a particular story from your life history – this could be from your personal or professional experience – and write it down. Please then answer the following questions:

- What made you think of that story?
- What feelings does the story bring back for you and why?
- Whose 'voices' appear in the story and what are your relationships and connections with them?
- What has changed between then and now, how has it changed and why might that be?
- Can you think of ways in which writing your autobiography might help develop your learning in terms of this story?

*There is some guidance on this activity at the end of the chapter.*

Autobiographical reflection also requires acknowledging how we feel about the past, and this may be difficult in terms of the emotional aspects that could appear or resurface. Nevertheless, being able to deal with your own emotions is one of the essential skills associated with being a nurse. The ability to acknowledge feelings and recognise what stimulates them, and why, is also a way of recognising our own humanity; this is an important aspect when entering a caring profession. This was emphasised in Chapter 1, in the story about Heather in Case Study 1.1, who worked in a learning disability community placement and highlighted uncaring behaviours that she felt did not recognise the humanity of others, interpreting these as possible reasons for care failings.

Remaining detached can be another way of coping, by suppressing feelings from past situations that are still active within the present. Cultural values are another rich stream that can be explored through autobiographical reflection, and this is looked at in more detail in Chapter 6.

Having explored what autobiographical reflection is, and having provided a few examples, we now consider how personal and professional experience might be integrated.

# Integrating personal and professional experience

Personal experience is a rich resource that may not always be seen as relevant to professional life, or professional experience. Nevertheless, as we have already mentioned, the skills and knowledge developed within personal experience are the foundation from which individuals develop their professional identity and skills. For example, some of the roles that we inhabit within our lives, such as being a child, sibling, parent, friend, neighbour, a member of a community group, and so on, bring valuable experiences that integrate with professional experience, to advance knowledge and practice in different ways, thereby enhancing knowledge and skills. Completing Activity 3.4 will help you to identify which different roles and experiences you can bring to that of being a (student) nurse.

## Activity 3.4 Reflection

Take some time to consider what roles you occupy in your personal life and the different activities in which you are involved. Write the things down as a list, as this will make them more tangible. You may be thinking of roles such as artist, activist, volunteer, carer, but these examples are not exhaustive and there are many others that could bring equally valuable experience. Bear in mind that the knowledge derived from the roles is dependent on the length of time you have been in the role, which transferable skills you have learned, and your degree of confidence to show and articulate your experiences.

Now consider how these roles might integrate with your professional life. Spend some time reflecting on the following questions. You may find this easier if you try to focus on one role at a time and work through all the questions before moving on to the next role.

- What knowledge is used in fulfilling the role? Where did you get this knowledge? Were you aware that you were learning this role? If so, provide some detail on this experience.
- Are any skills involved and, if so, what are they? How did you learn the skills? Were you aware of this learning? If so, write some detail on this experience.

- How might these skills be translated into different situations? In other words, think of examples where you have been able to use things that you have learned in one situation in a completely different situation.
- Where are there connections with the professional role?

*As this activity is based on your own experiences, there is no outline answer at the end of the chapter.*

Having completed Activity 3.4, you should now have a clearer idea of where to direct your reflection. Integrating personal and professional experience involves reflecting on what each contributes and how they relate to each other. It is worthwhile remembering that both personal and professional experiences feed into one result – shaping you (Buckley et al., 2024b). As previously mentioned, a change in one will automatically impact on the other. It is within integration that knowledge can be brought together as a whole or synthesised in more creative ways. For example, some of the knowledge developed through the parenting role is likely to include lifespan development, health management, communication and negotiation, leadership, organisation, nutrition, first aid and learning. Integration involves connecting this with what is learned through your professional role and, through reflecting imaginatively, identifying possibilities and ways of doing things.

As discussed in Chapter 1, imagining is part of a process of putting yourself into unknown situations and considering your actions and possible consequences. This might mean, when first entering the nursing programme or a new work environment, that you work from a position of personal experience and imagine how to respond to the situations discussed in class but have not yet experienced. 'Imagining' is a way of thinking about and questioning possibilities as part of development (Parse, 2004). Reflective imagining goes further by integrating the personal with the professional, identifying the required – and possibly ideal – response and what your likely response would be by using self-knowledge, and then thinking about what and how you could develop. This is clarified through reading Marc's biographical account in the Case Study below.

## Case Study 3.3: Marc's biographical account

Marc is French by birth but has been brought up in London since he was 7 years old. He is single and volunteers for a charity helpline in his spare time.

Marc is in the final year of his adult nursing apprentice programme. One of the more recent episodes of care that Marc wants to include in his e-portfolio is where he found he was able to integrate his personal and professional knowledge in a meaningful way.

Marc was on a community team placement. The team had been visiting a 24-year-old man, Pierre, daily to provide a wound dressing change. Pierre had been in a serious

*(Continued)*

(Continued)

road traffic accident in which his girlfriend had been fatally wounded. Pierre had needed a below-knee amputation of his left leg because of his injuries and had lost his job due to his immobility. Since his discharge from hospital, the wound on Pierre's stump had broken down and was taking a long time to heal. As it happened, Pierre was also French and spoke reasonable English but, over the weeks of visiting Pierre daily, Marc had noticed that he was becoming increasingly withdrawn.

Marc tried to imagine how Pierre must feel, losing so much so suddenly. Having previously written an essay on coping with grief and loss post-amputation, Marc knew that people often present with anxiety and depression, but he was uncertain how to approach this. Marc knew he had good communication skills from his charity helpline activity, but he was not a trained counsellor. He also knew that he could communicate in French with Pierre, which would be an advantage in helping Pierre to articulate his feelings. He started by checking his understanding of how Pierre was feeling but Marc soon realised that he did not have enough mental health knowledge to proceed further and suggested to his practice supervisor that a referral might be helpful.

Marc reflected on how often mental health and adult nursing issues overlapped. He considered that it would be good development, both professionally and personally, to undertake a counselling course. This experience helped him to recognise that, by integrating his personal and professional knowledge, he had been able to reach Pierre in a more personal way. With **reflexivity**, the experience had also shown him where he could develop further.

Marc's biographical account illustrates how reflective imagining begins when we are uncertain of what to do. Uncertainties in unknown situations can be disturbing. Jarvis (2007, p. 11) calls this *disharmony*. Although this might sound unacceptable, uncertainty is a normal part of critical thinking and, in fact, it is vital in helping us to set boundaries and decide whether to ask for help; it is crucial in how we risk assess situations and prompts the imagining referred to above. Connecting with others, reflecting and imagining are all part of critical thinking. Integrated thinking means acknowledging, firstly, that all experience can be useful to inform activity and, secondly, that different activities help to inform integrated thinking. However, thinking, as identified in Marc's account, can also create uncertainty and anxiety when we become aware of gaps in our knowledge. Reflection and imagining identify such gaps and can stimulate uncertainty and even anxiety. Identifying and acknowledging gaps in knowledge or skills allow us to undertake steps to resolve the gap; again, it helps us set clear boundaries in terms of our abilities and competence. As adults, and as professionals, situations of uncertainty stimulate us to look for solutions. These experiences can be drawn together through processes of self-reflection and through reflecting and imagining with others to expand our range of solutions. These processes, illustrated in Figure 3.1, represent how learning that integrates personal and professional experience might occur.

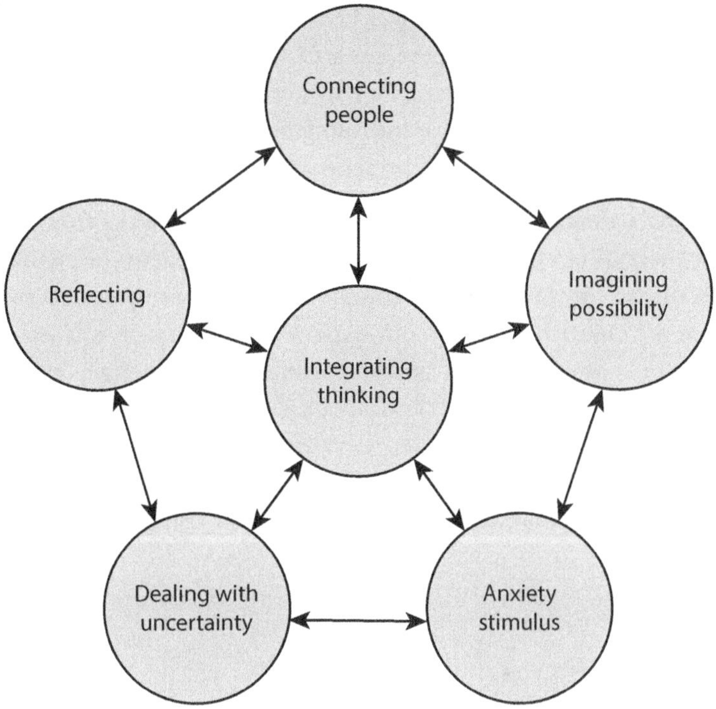


*Figure 3.1* Integration of personal and professional experience (from Howatson-Jones, 2010)

Integration is only possible when the processes of *disharmony* and accessing further information (including consulting others) have occurred. The reflective practitioner incorporates imagination to support new directions that take account of feedback. When all are completed, integrative thinking draws the parts together.

Integrative thinking uses meanings and symbolism. We first consider the meaning we give to a situation and communicate this with others. If our meaning is rejected, we may conform to their meaning as observed from their behaviour. Marc, in his account, checks his interpretation of how Pierre is feeling. When meaning is discussed, others' views are taken into consideration, and we use them to interpret the situation. Marc can identify that Pierre's feelings potentially translate into a mental health issue that needs addressing. Nevertheless, where others' interpretations become the accepted meaning, this may become fixed and conform to behavioural norms, for example, by viewing mental health and general nursing as something entirely separate. In this instance, Marc incorporates compassion, communication and courage, three of the 6 Cs: compassion by recognising Pierre's pain and possible feelings of guilt; communication by realising the importance of Pierre being able to talk and share his feelings, and possibly needing to do so in his own language; and courage by engaging in deeper interaction with Pierre without knowing what his response would be or whether Marc would be able to manage the responses, plus courage to decide to communicate in a language his colleague did not understand and taking the risk that the community nurse would feel excluded. Through his actions, Marc is addressing several important items in the section *Prioritise people* of the NMC Code (NMC, 2018b). By paying attention to Pierre's well-being and loss, and negotiating referral to mental health services,

Marc was addressing *Prioritise people* (items 3.1, 3.3, 3.4, 4.1, and 5.4) of the NMC's Code (NMC, 2018b). Marc's actions may seem obvious, but awareness of the actual situation prompts action from the nurse. By placing Pierre and his welfare centrally, applying the 6 Cs and being aware of personal strengths and limitations, Marc can make the appropriate decisions and meet the standards of the profession.

We manage anxiety by determining whether conforming behaviours (for example, ideas of peers, supervisors, lecturers, etc.) restrict our reflective imagination or enable us to develop ideas and reach out to the unknown. Throughout the process we need to be aware and reflect on how we are changing through our experiences. Although uncomfortable, anxiety stimulates us to think of alternatives and experiment with change, but it needs to be accompanied by self-awareness to overcome any obstacles that restrict positive progress. For example, Marc's confidence has increased because his practice supervisor has taken his concern seriously. These points are illustrated in Figure 3.2. The influence of anxiety is shown at the crossing points marked with an X and the arrows represent potential direction.

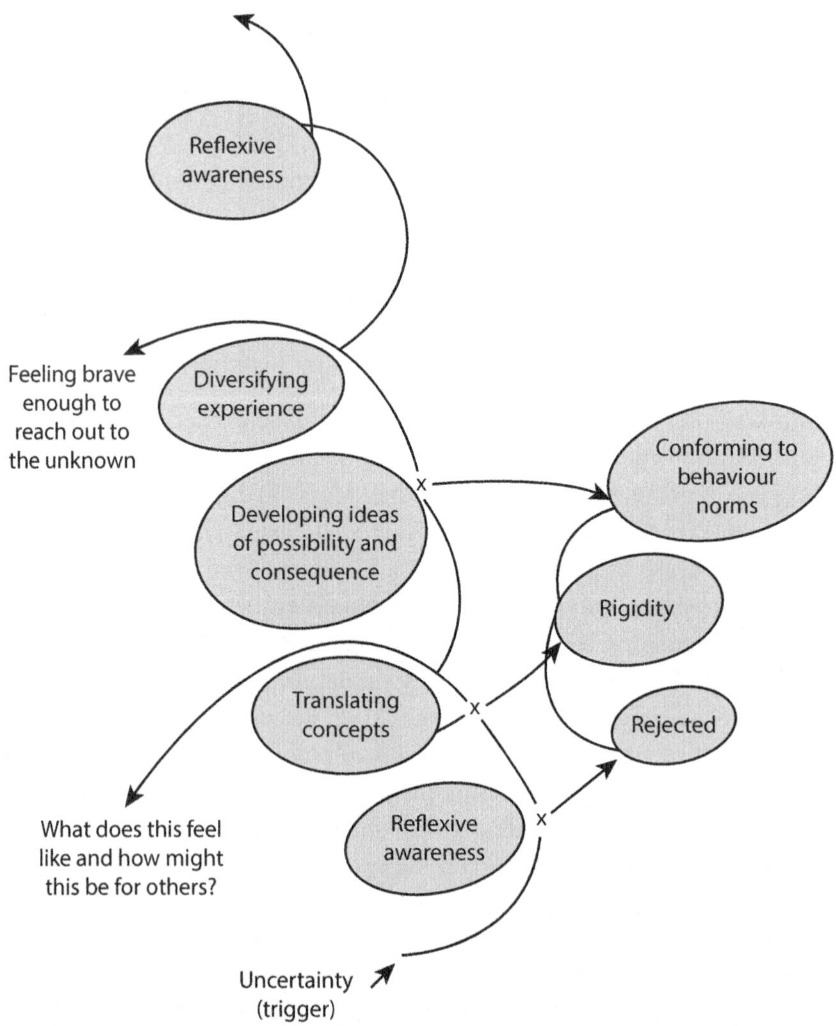


*Figure 3.2* Schema of reflective imagination (from Howatson-Jones, 2010)

Review your own meaning making and development of ideas by completing Activity 3.5.

### Activity 3.5 Critical thinking

- Looking back on your own life, identify a situation where you were anxious and uncertain of how to proceed, or where you were moving into a new beginning. You might consider when you were starting your nursing programme, your first day on a new placement or moving into your first qualified role after completing the programme.
- Reflect on how you made meaning of the situation. By using the schema in Figure 3.2, can you see where you might have been conforming to behavioural norms or, alternatively, where meaning is coming from developing ideas and reflexive awareness?

*There is an outline answer to this activity at the end of the chapter.*

Now that you have identified experiences from your own life and considered how you developed meaning and following on from what you have learned so far about autobiographical reflection and integrating personal and professional experiences, we move to a life story exercise that helps you to prepare your autobiography.

### Activity 3.6 Reflection

Compile a written account of your life story so far. This might include aspects such as:

- where you were born;
- family, siblings, parents, extended family;
- friends growing up and friends later in life;
- growing up;
- significant events;
- school;
- first job;
- choice of career;
- interests.

*As this activity relates to your own experience, there is no outline answer at the end of the chapter.*

It helps to write your autobiography in the chronological order in which things happened. You may not remember everything at once, so go back and add things as you remember them. It is helpful to select a personal photograph or a picture from a magazine that symbolises how you view the world and then discuss the item by describing why it is important to you and how it represents your story. Illustrate the aspects you have chosen to include with examples. In talking about specific events, try to focus on their meaning as well as their factual content but always remember confidentiality.

### Activity 3.7 Reflection

When you have completed the account, think about the following questions:

- How did constructing your autobiography make you feel?
- Whose voices appear in the construction? For example, you may find that an aspect that you feel strongly about comes directly from someone else. Is this then your voice, or theirs? Perhaps you realise that you have developed a very different idea to what you were brought up to believe. How does this realisation make you feel?
- How do you regulate emotion?
- Did you have any concerns and, if so, what were these?
- Are there elements you wish to change and, if so, why?
- What might this process tell you about working with and caring for people?

*As this activity relates to your own experience, there is no outline answer at the end of the chapter.*

This exercise aims to help you to be aware of your personal values and develop your professional values. For example, think about how you are developing the 6 Cs in your way of being. Having asked you to compile your autobiography, we now consider how you can examine and reflect on its content to develop your learning.

## How to examine and reflect upon autobiography

You will have taken time to decide what to include in your autobiography and such decisions will be influenced by the purpose of writing it. While the exercise in this book requests you to write your autobiography, remember that you are doing it for yourself, so consider what your purpose is for undertaking the activity. Your writing may be affected by who the potential readers are and the range of experiences you must choose from. All these aspects are of interest when starting to analyse your autobiography.

The way you structure your autobiography can convey a sense of how your experiences have shaped you and, at the same time, it could also be a process of repair and change where experiences have been difficult or painful (Fischer-Rosenthal, 2000). By examining your autobiography, you develop self-awareness, and reflecting upon it is a way to influence future direction actively and initiate change.

It takes time and effort to properly examine and reflect on your autobiography. This starts from the time of constructing it and continues through to its completion and beyond. This process is part of a life-long activity and is, consequently, ongoing. Understanding what you need to learn, and accessing sources to achieve this, is an essential part of life-long learning. You are encouraged to return to your autobiography periodically to understand and be aware of your development through questioning context, feelings and knowledge base – all of which are important features in any type of reflection. To gain true personal and professional development we also need to focus on connections between experiences past, present and future, and examine ways in which thinking has changed or is changing, and what our personal responses to this are. Another important aspect to consider includes the regulation of emotion in terms of how it is shown, by examining different 'voices' and emerging themes (Horsdal, 2012). This allows us to look at what is being internalised and how this occurs. This might seem to be quite a difficult activity to undertake, but this level of reflection helps us become resilient and develop the ability to manage issues and challenges that we face along the way. The *Promote professionalism and trust* section of the NMC's Code (2018b) addresses the importance of being aware of how our behaviour can impact others (item 20.3) and the importance of maintaining an optimal level of health (item 20.9). These items resonate with Jen's story, where stress and disappointment could have an impact on how she approaches her learning and patient care. We all face challenging situations throughout our lives, but we need to build resilience to manage ourselves appropriately; this type of reflection allows us to build this resilience and is part of being a professional.

Case Study 3.4, Jen's biographical account, is provided to illustrate significant features that may be relevant to past, present and future learning and associated emotional aspects. You are asked to identify some of these features after reading the scenario.

## Case Study 3.4: Jen's biographical account

Jen is in the second semester of the first year of her mental health nursing programme after completing her A levels. Having grown up in a small town, she now enjoys the hustle and bustle of city living. She particularly enjoys the freedom of living away from home, but finds the more independent mode of study, when compared with school, challenging.

Jen grew up in a close-knit family and is the middle child of three. Her family has lived in the same place for as long as Jen can remember, and she has always been very close to her maternal grandmother who lived nearby. Visiting her paternal grandparents was an annual holiday treat because they lived some hours away at the coast.

Jen had always wanted to be a nurse because she saw herself being able to 'do good' and 'care for other people'. Jen's parents were supportive and encouraged her to go into nursing because of the job security that the education could provide, and

*(Continued)*

(Continued)

they considered it a 'noble profession'. They were, however, apprehensive of their daughter moving 'so far away' and being the first in the family to go to university. Finance was another point of concern, but, as Jen had obtained particularly good A levels, they felt that they did not want to stand in their daughter's way.

Jen had recently received her first assignment grade of a borderline pass and was finding her first assessed placement particularly challenging. These two elements have left her feeling quite despondent and doubting her capabilities. She really wants to return home to be with her parents and grandmother but knows that she cannot miss any of the placement time. Besides, she needs to be mindful of finances because she has spent too much money already when socialising with her new friends.

## Activity 3.8 Identifying

- What are the significant features within this biographical account and why? Think particularly about what may be relevant to Jen's past, present, and future learning and her associated emotional needs.

*There is an outline answer to this question at the end of the chapter.*

Having read Jen's biographical account and answered the question at the end, you will be able to see that examining and reflecting are not the same. Examining your autobiography means collating events and looking for particular features. It also means paying attention to the factual content. This might include questions such as the following:

- What is the timeline of events? Identifying the timeline gives clues to the different stages of your life and how these might relate to external events.
- What decisions were made? Decision-making can provide information about how you were thinking at the time.
- How is identity visible? Is there a difference between role and identity? Tracing the thread of an identity helps to raise awareness of changes and the circumstances that affect this. Do different roles call for different identities? What would this mean for you?
- Where is learning evident? Identifying learning helps to develop personal knowledge. Again, does this knowledge help you develop an identity or a particular role?

Examining your autobiography also requires you to ask more contemplative questions about the relationships between people and the construction of the story. For example, what underlies the direction and focus of the construction of your story and its inclusions? This helps in reflecting on more hidden meanings.

It is by reflecting on your autobiographical account that you can make sense from it in distinguishing between then and now, and how meaning is constantly evolving in the light of new knowledge, the connections made, strategies identified and learning taken forward. Equally, reflecting on the features within it starts to reveal changes in your role and your (professional) identity as you develop. For example, think of your identity and role as a child and then as an adult. Although your role as a child or sibling has remained unchanged within the family, your identity has developed and, as a result, your perception of your role has altered. Your changed perception has changed the dynamics within the family structure, and, through the change, you have 'demanded' that others within the family view you differently. These changes can clearly be seen during puberty. Such development can be called a process of **becoming**. Similarly, as the novice professional grows in skill and knowledge of what it is to be a professional (identity), so the perceptions of the role change and develop (McClunie-Trust et al., 2025; Sherwood, 2024). Initially reflecting on the new role may include the following questions:

- Which elements from your personal history give this event significance? Look back across your life experience and review what is active. Taking note of the experiences is one way to start making the connections from which new insights emerge.
- What meaning does this have? Making sense of new insights requires defining what we mean.
- What did the environment or context contribute to this meaning? Contexts encompass objects, people, cultures and society, all of which influence behaviour and the meaning we give things.
- How do I feel about this now? Reviewing how feelings change helps to acknowledge and make sense of emotional learning and the associated development of your thinking.
- How is my identity changing? Reviewing a changing identity helps to develop self-awareness and reflexivity in how events are shaping you as a person and as a professional.
- Do you respond differently if you are expected to do something beyond your competence as a professional or if you are confronted by inappropriate behaviour? Reviewing where your boundaries lie and how you establish and maintain your boundaries is an important element of professional development.
- Are my values changing or have they changed? Reviewing changes in values can provide clues about societal or cultural influences that are instrumental in shaping you as a professional.

However, contemplative reflection also requires asking broader questions about the role we take in shaping our world and the role of the world in shaping us. For example, a person who has come from another country, or perhaps another region, will have an identity that is rooted in the cultural values of that place. The starting point is to reflect on what these might be in the first instance, to be able to identify a change and where that then stems from – whether from the person or perhaps a necessity to conform. An example you may want to reflect on would be the choices an individual may need to make in accepting and coming out in terms of sexual orientation or gender identity (See Pippa's case study (Case Study 2.2).

Now use these suggestions to examine and reflect on your autobiography to complete Activity 3.8.

### Activity 3.9 Critical thinking

Examine and reflect on your own autobiography, which you compiled earlier, using the suggestions above and the following questions:

- What does your autobiography contribute to your learning to be a professional?
- What potential alternative strategies does your autobiography contribute to your learning and decision-making?
- What conclusions have you reached from this exercise?
- What new insights have you developed and why?

*There is an outline answer to this activity at the end of the chapter.*

Having asked you to examine and reflect on your own autobiography, we now consider how this relates to our perception of societal issues.

# Identifying subjective perception of societal issues

Developing an autobiography can help us illustrate issues that are/were present in society at that time, and how they affect us through having a lived experience of the issues. This is one way in which an autobiography raises awareness of social processes as in West's work (2001). In healthcare, professionals need to be conscious of the uniqueness of each person's **lived experience** and the services they have accessed, but at the same time remain aware of how an individual health experiences contribute to a wider understanding of health issues. Queens nurses reflect well on how this is achieved here https://qicn.org.uk/voice-and-value/nurses-stories/.

Consider this example, an experience of unemployment you have had may reveal how welfare is organised, and thought of, within societal structures. Such experiences may even change your previously held views and social values and the power of the message imparted through your subjective experience could have far-reaching and life-long effects. This creates a lens through which social issues and others' experiences can be perceived.

Critically reflecting on subjective experience is a way to (1) acknowledge its value in developing understanding and (2) reveal how personal views may have become shaped by others and become entrenched as norms. What is perceived as normal and helpful through childhood experiences may be viewed very differently when looking back more critically from adult experience (Brookfield, 2005). Such critical reflection looks back and examines issues of power surrounding events and the learning taken from them. The following Case Study of subjective perception of societal issues provides an illustration of such a process.

## Case Study 3.5: Identifying subjective perception of societal issues

Kelly is in the third year of my adult apprentice nurse programme. This year, the focus of the modules she is undertaking is on developing skills in leadership, managing care and making the transition into practice. Her previous placement as on a surgical ward where she managed the care of several women. One patient, Jane, was of concern and Kelly reflected critically on the situation, which has led her to question personal values and those of society.

Kelly admitted Jane for an excision biopsy of suspected breast cancer. Jane also had learning disabilities and so attended with her carer. Kelly was surprised by this as she has a brother with learning disabilities who lives with the family and goes to a mainstream school. Kelly started to admit Jane by talking to her directly, but her carer intervened, answering on her behalf. She then completed Jane's admission and started to prepare her for the procedure. Clearly Jane was frightened and confused by what was happening, so Kelly took some time to sit with her and explain what was happening. She used drawings to show Jane what she needed to communicate when it became apparent that Jane did not understand, and she did the same thing when the surgeon and anaesthetist came to see Jane. Kelly accompanied Jane to theatre and collected her after the procedure to ensure that she saw a familiar face.

When reflecting on this incident, some insights came to Kelly. She realised that she sees the person, rather than the condition. However, she noted the surgeon and anaesthetist's limited response when faced by Jane's lack of understanding. Kelly began to wonder whether the voices of people with a learning disability are always heard by those caring for them. On reflection she realised that her values and beliefs in seeing the person rather than a diagnosis were based on her lived experience with her brother. She assumed that these values are more mainstream because her brother's school friends accepted him as he is.

Kelly could see the difficulties exist within certain institutions, such as the hospital, and reflected on whether these difficulties stem from a society that is less comfortable with difference and does not, therefore, offer appropriate provision according to person-centred need, but rather according to deficit. Kelly thought about why her values are different. Having grown up with her brother and knowing him and his ways, would she find his outbursts frightening if she did not know him?

*(Continued)*

(Continued)

She wondered how much of this is related to control. Is a **deficit model** a kind of control? Kelly realised that control comes in many forms, not least in building relationships.

In this case study, Kelly has identified disharmony between her taken-for-granted values and those she is experiencing in her student nurse role. This has led her to reflect on why societal values might differ from hers and to question her assumptions. From such a position Kelly can advocate more effectively for those in her care by entering the societal debate more knowledgeably. You are advised to find items from the NMC's Code (2018b) that relate to Kelly's situation, for example, in the sections *Prioritise people* (items 1.1, 1.3, 1.5, 2.1–2.4, 2.6, and 3.4) and *Promote professionalism* (items 20.5 and 20.7). Please complete Activity 3.10 to identify some of your own values and assumptions.

## Activity 3.10 Critical thinking

Can you think of experiences in your own life that have helped to develop your understanding of some social issues? Reflect on these by looking at the following questions. To help you with this activity, you may want to consider the 'protected characteristics' (Equality Act 2010) as a starting point.

- What were the assumptions surrounding the situation?
- What values were active in the situation?
- What did you learn about the social issue?
- Has anything changed because of this learning?

*There is an outline answer to this activity at the end of the chapter.*

By identifying your own assumptions and values through the activity and reflecting on the learning you have achieved in the situations you reflected on, you may be able to be a more effective advocate for those in your care in similar circumstances.

## Chapter summary

This chapter explains the ways in which autobiography contributes to learning as a professional. By offering several suggestions of how to compile, examine and reflect on a personal biography, the chapter provided the starting and developing healthcare professional with the possibility of integrating personal and professional experiences into something meaningful to their learning. In this way, it becomes possible to understand personal learning needs and objectives better, develop professional values and recognise a developing (professional) identity.

## Brief outline answers

In this section, answers to the chapter's activities will be outlined and explained.

### Activity 3.1 Reflection

The learning Callum may have taken forward is:

- Formal learning can be painful and confusing.
- It is difficult to trust and feel comfortable with peers.
- It is important to be helpful and caring to be accepted by others.

### Activity 3.2 Reflection

The meaning that Callum is likely to have attached is the following:

- Learning at school was a struggle.
- He can inspire others.
- He can trust people to support him.
- Asking for help can be difficult.
- It is difficult to trust that others will provide support.
- Asking for support can be a good thing.

Some creative strategies that Callum could employ might be:

- to focus on trying to articulate the subjects he needs to learn, as if he were motivating a rugby team;
- to realise that everyone has their strengths and role to play within a group;
- to try to break down the task he needs to learn into smaller parts and understand what support he needs to be successful;
- to work with others as study partners;
- to use his sense of tactics to plan his learning and manage his time;
- to talk things over with lecturers and practice supervisors;
- to be open and honest with colleagues, lecturers, and practice supervisors.

### Activity 3.3 Critical thinking

Your answer may have related to the following key points:

- recognising important relationships;
- acknowledging emotional blocks and drivers in learning;
- developing understanding of strengths and areas of development;
- developing self-knowledge.

### Activity 3.5 Critical thinking

When thinking about first starting the nurse preparation programme or moving into practice, you may have included:

- needing to identify what was expected by your practice supervisor and practice colleagues or by the regulatory body;
- professional behaviours;
- knowledge base.

When considering integrating thinking, you may have included:

- fitting into the team and learning what it means to be a healthcare professional;
- working interprofessionally to gain a wider perspective;

- reflecting on reasons for anxiety and uncertainty and addressing knowledge gaps;
- integrating reflective and imaginative ideas.

## Activity 3.8 Identifying

This scenario includes the following features, which provide a good starting point for further examination and reflection on what is brought to the nursing course and how this is progressing:

- moving from a town to a new city;
- changing study experiences;
- enjoying social processes;
- loss of parental and family support networks;
- teaching and leadership skills;
- being responsible and accountable for actions and choices;
- self-reliance.

## Activity 3.9 Critical thinking

You may have addressed this activity by considering difficult events, how the past has been overcome and how you are taking something forward into the future in a more positive way. Or you may have used a cautionary tale of how not to proceed, or a moral story of the right thing to do. Reflection may have included looking at emotional as well as cognitive learning, and how your identity is developing.

## Activity 3.10 Critical thinking

Answers to the activity are likely to have centred around:

- values such as dignity and respect, person-centredness, compassion, and holistic care;
- assumptions;
- societal views;
- learning.

# Further reading

**Buckley, A. R. & Corless, L.** (2025). The PRISM model: A new framework for interpreting health narratives. *Nursing Times, 121*(11).

**Buckley, A. R., Corless, L., Crowle, A., Gallacher, J. & Watkinson, K.** (2024a). Narratives: A powerful tool in nurse education and practice. *Nursing Times, 120*(9).

**Buckley, A. R., Corless, L., Taylor, A., Warren, E. & May, F.** (2024b). Speaking up for patients: Advocacy and narrative work in nursing. *Nursing Times, 120*(11).

These are a series of exemplary reflective articles presented by nursing students about the people in their care and indicate how to reflect well.

**Horsdal, M.** (2012). *Telling lives: Exploring dimensions of narratives.* Routledge.

This book identifies the relevance and importance of how we construct our biographies to tell others who we are and why we respond in certain ways.

**Price, B.** (2025). *Delivering person-centred care in nursing* (3rd ed.). Sage/Learning Matters.

This book emphasises the importance of eliciting and reflecting on patient narratives to enhance person-centred care.

## Useful websites

**https://www.nice.org.uk/guidance/ng240**

This guideline covers recognising, diagnosing and managing bacterial meningitis and meningococcal disease in babies, children, young people and adults.

**https://qicn.org.uk/voice-and-value/nurses-stories/**

These are a selection of rich stories from Queens Nurses in the community.

**https://www.youtube.com/watch?v=hjYYOItV-44**

**https://www.youtube.com/watch?v=nxfNSJ47LZo**

**https://www.youtube.com/watch?v=2hOgN0tRscs**

Examples of autobiographical reflections, nursing, teaching and art.

# Chapter 4 Reflective models and frameworks

## NMC Future Nurse: Standards of Proficiency for Registered Nurses

This chapter will address the following platforms and proficiencies:

**Platform 1: Being an accountable professional**

1.17 Take responsibility for continuous self-reflection, seeking and responding to support and feedback to develop their professional knowledge and skills.

**Platform 5: Leading and managing nursing care and working in teams**

5.10 Contribute to supervision and team reflection activities to promote improvements in practice and services.

**Platform 6: Improving safety and quality of care**

6.12 Understand the role of registered nurses and other health and care professionals at different levels of experience and seniority when managing and prioritising actions and care in the event of a major incident.

## Chapter aims

After reading this chapter you will be able to:

- identify different models and frameworks of reflection;
- consider strengths and limitations of different models and frameworks;
- choose an appropriate model or framework for your reflection.

## Case Study 4.1: Jane's use of empathy

Jane was placed in a surgical outpatient department as a second-year nurse apprentice. She noticed Sarah in the waiting area who appeared emotional and nervous. As Jane had received feedback in her first year that she needed to be proactive in engaging with the people coming into her care, she introduced herself to Sarah, who was in her early 30s. Sarah was waiting to see the consultant about a lump in her left breast. After discussing it with her practice supervisor, James, Jane asked Sarah if she could sit in on her consultation. Sarah agreed, becoming quite tearful.

During the examination, the consultant asked Sarah what she thought the lump could be, at which point Sarah began to cry. She disclosed she thought that she might have cancer as the lump had been there for some time and her grandmother had died from metastatic breast cancer. Jane found this situation difficult; she wanted to put her arm around Sarah and comfort her. However, she felt 'outside' the communication bubble between Sarah and her consultant. Jane made the decision only to observe. The consultant listened to Sarah's concerns and calmly explained that this was one possibility, but that there were other causes of a breast lump. He suggested completing the necessary tests before reaching a conclusion. He went on to explain the tests to Sarah but quickly realised that Sarah appeared not to be processing the information. He asked Jane to give Sarah some refreshment and go through the relevant patient information leaflets to help her assimilate the information. He then saw his next patient. Jane sat with Sarah as she tried to read the leaflets and offered to help Sarah write down any questions she had. The consultant then saw Sarah again to answer her questions. Jane was surprised by a second consultation in what was a busy clinic. At the end of the shift, she discussed her day with James and said that she had not seen a doctor be as unhurried and interested with someone, even though there had been a full list of people to see. James suggested that Jane reflect on the differences she had noticed in the way this consultant worked and what the potential outcomes might be for those in his care, the staff and the organisation.

That evening Jane spent time reflecting on her day. She began by thinking about how she had seen other healthcare professionals interact with the people in their care and the differences she had noticed with this consultant. She noted that the consultant was completely focused on Sarah and was not trying to write or look at the computer or notes at the same time. She also noted that he had attentively listened to Sarah's concerns about the lump and had given her time to absorb his explanation and to ask further questions. Jane associated this situation with her own experience of having a cervical smear test, not understanding the results, and feeling frustrated that no one appeared to be listening to her or explain what they were doing. She wondered whether the consultant had experienced being a service

*(Continued)*

(Continued)

user himself or if he had experienced similar situations with family members that might explain his actions.

Jane thought of what the outcome for Sarah would be, feeling that her concerns had been listened to. Jane imagined that staff would find the consultant as approachable as she had, and that the organisation would benefit from such a collegiate, interprofessional atmosphere contributing to a positive workplace culture. Jane thought about what she was taking forward from this reflection and decided it was the realisation of how important attentive listening is to good person centred care. She discussed her reflections with James the next day; he agreed and added that focusing on the positives of the situation would enable her to use this approach within her practice.

The next day, in the waiting room, Jane observed Mrs Scott, an older woman looking anxiously at the clock while she waited for her dermatology appointment. She tentatively approached Mrs Scott and began a conversation. Jane tried to focus on listening attentively and not to look too pointedly at the skin discolouration on Mrs Scott's arms, hands, arm and neck. Jane was aware of thinking that they looked quite uncomfortable and thought of how embarrassed she would be if she had a condition that was so visible to others. One of the first things that Mrs Scott said was that her husband had dementia, that she was his primary carer and that she was anxious to get back home. Jane shared this information during the consultation as she observed that the consultation had, until then, been focused purely on physical results. This resulted in the consultant being able to consider stress as a potential underlying cause of Mrs Scott's symptoms.

## Activity 4.1 Reflection

Imagine yourself in Jane's position or recall a similar experience. Write down the scenario. Then, consider the following questions:

- What goes through your mind when you are with someone of a similar age who is distressed?
- How do you feel in this situation? Are your thoughts and emotions similar or different?
- Reflect on your behaviour. Were you influenced by your thoughts and emotions? Did you become emotional or distant? Was this professional behaviour? Why?
- Do you respond the same way with someone older than yourself? Why or why not? Consider your examples in terms of 'person-centred care'.

*As this is a reflective exercise for yourself, there is no outline answer at the end of the chapter.*

This reflective exercise demonstrates how situations that arouse emotions can stimulate thinking about them. Use your examples further along in this chapter where you will work through them using reflective cycles, to help demonstrate different stages of a reflective process. Using models and reflective cycles can help you, especially if you are less experienced, develop your reflection into something that enables you to examine your learning fully.

# Introduction

This chapter introduces some of the wide range of reflective models and frameworks that you can draw from when first starting, to structure and frame your reflections. You are encouraged to consider some of the strengths and limitations of the **reflective frameworks**, models and cycles, to help you to choose appropriately. The right questions to ask will be highlighted through the example and case study presented.

# Reflective frameworks

Donald Schön (1991) examined how professionals think about what they are doing and described these ways of thinking as reflection-in-action and reflection-on-action. When in a situation, we are constantly reworking problems and discovering consequences from this reworking, and these have implications for further adaptations. Schön (1991) identifies this as a framing process whereby, through reframing roles and perspectives of a situation, new phenomena come into view and can be worked in other ways that may bring different solutions. In the example, Jane observes a positive communication style that she recognises as contrasting with the pressured version with which she is more familiar. By recognising the benefits for the patient, the organisation and herself, and using her analysis to reframe her future communications, Jane reflects on how her attitude and communication could allow her to contribute effectively to the workplace. This is often known as reflection-before-action and Jane had this in mind when she tentatively approached Mrs Scott. It was quite understandable for Jane to feel a little apprehensive when approaching a service user initially. In starting a conversation with Mrs Scott, Jane would become aware of how Mrs Scott communicated with her: her intonation, non-verbal communication and choice of words. Naturally, Jane would not know which direction the interaction would take but, using the cues she received from Mrs Scott and the communication theory she had covered, Jane felt that she would have been able to respond appropriately to Mrs Scott's concerns. Reflection-in-action can, therefore, be described as a form of experimentation in problem-solving that acknowledges uncertainty and looks at discovering potential answers or ways to proceed. Schön (1991, p. 76) describes this as having a *reflective conversation with the situation*, which is also the strength of this approach, in that it is working with the situation in real time. In other words, we are constantly interpreting and responding to cues within the situation and consequently changing its course in the process. Nevertheless, a limitation is that much of this reflection often occurs unconsciously as part of working with experience intuitively. 'Intuitively' means that articulated descriptions can never fully explain the actions taken or knowledge used, or artistry involved (Schön, 1991, p. 276). Undertaking Activity 4.2 will help you to understand these points.

## Activity 4.2 Evidence-based practice and reflection

Observe someone undertaking an activity. It may be your practice supervisor on placement or a lecturer in class. If you are an experienced practitioner, it may be an advanced practitioner in their field. Consider how their activity flows and whether they seem to be aware of each process or step they are undertaking. For example, think about the following.

- When is it obvious to you that they have in some way modified their actions?
- Were there hesitations when they might have thought about what they were doing and altered direction?
- What happened when you, or somebody else, asked them a question?
- How was the answer worked out?

*There is an outline answer to this activity at the end of the chapter.*

The process of reflection-in-action enables adaptation of learning from experience during action. Critical analysis, which will be explored as critical reflection in more detail in Chapter 11, helps to formalise and record these processes. When completing nursing activities, you may have become aware that you are not conscious of thoughts at the time, but that you are responding to what you think the situation might require. This is because, when we stop, we become more aware of what is going on in our thinking as well as acting. We also become conscious of what we have learnt through the action we have undertaken, when looking back on it. Schön (1991) suggests that thinking too much about action while undertaking it might raise barriers to the smooth flow of the action. Although you may feel that thinking about your every move limits your activity, you might want to bear in mind that, when learning new skills or activities, it is completely normal that you need to think through each step. You will find that, as you gain experience, you will be able to think things through (reflection-in-action) at the same time as undertaking the activity. However, equally beneficial to your learning is to look back at the action. This can help professionals gain greater insight and clarity in their thought processes and the actions taken. This is called reflection-on-action. As seen in Case Study 4.1 the process of reflection-on-action highlights the learning achieved for future use and is particularly useful for the novice to undertake. Completing Activity 4.3 may help you to identify some of your own learning from reflection-on-action.

### Activity 4.3 Critical thinking

Reflect on Case Study 4.1 and answer the following questions:

- What was the patient's issue?
- Was the issue clear from the start?
- Were there different interpretations of the issue?
- How did these interpretations become clear?
- Were you aware of these interpretations during the situation?
- What discoveries did you make?
- How did these discoveries influence your actions?
- How did your actions address the problem?
- What did you learn from the situation?

Now consider a recent patient-related situation when you worked with your practice supervisor or, if you are an experienced practitioner, think of a time when you worked with a student. Consider a patient-related issue that you encountered together and consider the earlier questions again.

*There is an outline answer to this activity at the end of the chapter.*

As you completed Activity 4.3 you may have become aware of elements in the activity that were, perhaps, not obvious to you at the time, or you may have identified gaps in your knowledge. In the next section we consider how using a reflective model can help you to question some of these elements to develop your learning and to question the evidence base that supports what you are doing.

## Reflective models

Reflection requires some effort and practice to maintain the necessary focus on thoughts, feelings and memories for making appropriate changes (Taylor, 2010). For example, you may find it emotionally difficult when dealing with death and dying. It is often useful to use a model because it will help you to maintain focus and identify key stages of your reflective learning. The structure of a model can provide you with foundations that help you to keep going when you are managing complex issues and to arrive at a resolution about how to deal with the situation. It is important to choose a model that suits your needs and that you find easy to use. Nevertheless, for reflection to be of value and to maintain progression in your life-long learning, it is important to reflect on what you are doing regularly and on your learning. In fact, we should all strive to embed reflection as an integral part of who we are as learners and practitioners. In other words, reflection should become a way of being – second nature – rather than something that you do as an add-on or because you need to include it in an assignment.

In Chapter 1, we referred to Barksby et al. (2015), who suggest a new model of reflection for clinical practice, but we also suggested that this 'new' approach is built on earlier, seminal models. It is highly beneficial to have some understanding of the development of reflective thinking to nursing and the following models offer several perspectives, areas on which to focus your reflection and questions you might want to ask yourself. The principles of the models are similar, and they all provide a framework and cue questions to support reflective thinking, so try to be selective when choosing a model to work with because, besides personal preference, the situation and context could lend themselves better to one model rather than another.

Johns (2025) has developed and refined the following model over several years through working with many practitioners at different stages of their development. This is an important point to realise: reflection is dynamic and the ways in which it is undertaken are constantly evolving. Therefore, any model can only ever be a guide rather than being a final template for reflection.

## Model for structured reflection

The Model for Structured Reflection (MSR; Johns, 2025) identifies how you might examine your experience more extensively and in greater depth to really learn from it. The model's starting point is to create space for reflection – what Johns (2025) calls *bringing the mind home*, so you can focus. The model then encompasses several reflective cues, or questions, which the practitioner is asked to think about while reflecting on a situation. These are presented below.

### Concept summary: MSR reflective cues

- Bringing the mind home.
- Description of positive and problematic issues.
- Reflection on what occurred in terms of the following:
    - What issues are significant to pay attention to?
    - How were others feeling and why did they feel that way?
    - How was I feeling and what made me feel that way?
    - What was I trying to achieve, and did I respond effectively?
    - What were the consequences of my actions on the patient, others and myself?
    - To what extent did I act for the best and in tune with my values?
    - What knowledge did or might have informed me?
    - How does this situation connect with previous experiences?
    - What assumptions govern my practice and what factors influence the way I feel, think and respond to the situation?

*Anticipation in terms of:*

- How might I reframe the situation to respond more effectively?
- What would be the consequences of responding differently for the patient, others and myself?
- What factors might constrain me responding in new ways?
- How do I feel about this experience now?

*Insights in terms of:*

- What insights have I gained? (framing perspectives)

(*Source*: Johns, 2013)

These cues encompass aesthetic, personal, ethical, empirical and reflexive aspects that are related to Carper's (1978) fundamental patterns of knowing (Johns, 1995):

- Aesthetics relates to how the person feels about, responds to and perceives the situation and those involved.
- Personal aspects explore, from the person, what was influencing them.
- Ethics encompasses how actions are related to beliefs.
- Empirics is concerned with what knowledge was used.
- Reflexivity relates to how experiences are connected and the possible alternatives and changes to doing things differently.

The following case study makes use of these cues to help illustrate how this model might be applied.

## Case Study 4.2: Tamara's experience of comforting

Tamara was working on a gynaecology ward as a trainee nursing associate and her practice supervisor had arranged for her to spend some time in the early pregnancy unit with the scanning nurse, Pip. Pip scanned a woman called Monica and found that there was no foetal heartbeat. When she informed Monica of this, she was understandably very upset. Pip asked Tamara to stay with Monica while she made further arrangements.

Tamara took Monica to a room where they could talk privately as she thought that Monica would appreciate the space to express her feelings. Monica began to cry, and Tamara said that it was okay for Monica to express her feelings. Tamara sat close to Monica, to give her some comfort, but not touching. She was not sure how Monica would react to a stranger as Tamara herself did not like strangers touching her. Tamara allowed Monica to cry for a while and then asked her if she wanted anyone to be contacted. Monica said she did not want to disturb her partner at work. She asked why her baby had died; Tamara explained that she was a trainee and would get Pip. At that moment Pip came into the room to explain the next steps. She told Monica that the reasons for foetal death are often not known, and further tests would be carried out.

*(Continued)*

(Continued)

Later that day Tamara's link tutor, Lynne, came to the ward. It was obvious to Lynne that Tamara was upset, so they accessed quiet area to talk privately. Tamara told Lynne about her morning and she felt that she should have done more but was not sure what, this had upset her. Lynne helped Tamara to reflect on the situation. They identified that Tamara had used a person-centred approach by offering Monica privacy and giving her time to express her feelings. Tamara had not imposed her own views on the situation and had sought help when asked questions that were outside her sphere of knowledge. Lynne asked Tamara what she had learnt from the situation. Tamara said that the overriding thing she had learnt was that we do not always have answers. She felt she could perhaps have done more to comfort Monica. Lynne and Tamara explored the options of using touch. Lynne advised Tamara to revisit communication literature. Tamara felt less upset and decided that next time, she would talk to her practice supervisor about the situation. Nevertheless, she felt she had handled a difficult situation well.

The case study illustrates how reflection can also affirm actions as well as correct them. Using this model helps to expose how others might be thinking and how to approach this. It is an important point to consider in more depth. Often, we reflect on situations that have not gone well or where we think that there could be room for improvement. Although this is, undoubtedly, important, we should remember that most of what we do is of good quality, achieves appropriate outcomes and those in our care are satisfied. It is, therefore, also important to reflect on things that have gone well because these situations offer cues as to what works successfully and what our strengths are and, consequently, allows us to develop a broad range of 'tried and tested' approaches to situations. One might say that this is how we build our **intuition** but the strength in this would arguably be our ability to make conscious use of in-, on- or before-action reflection.

## Stages of reflection

We move on now to consider another model by Atkins and Murphy (1995), which examines three main stages to reflection based on feelings, knowledge and coming to new ways of thinking.

- Stage 1: awareness of uncomfortable feelings.
- Stage 2: critical analysis of the situation.
- Stage 3: development of new perspectives on the situation.

Stage 1 of this model relates to uncomfortable feelings as the stimulus for starting to reflect on what is causing them and what can be done. Part of this will be an assessment of your knowledge base and whether this was sufficient. Atkins and Murphy (1995) make the point here that feelings need not necessarily be negative but can be more positively related to some achievement. It may be useful to qualify this point with reference to Jarvis

(2007, p. 3), who describes such a state as 'disharmony'. This occurs when there is a break with familiar experience that alerts the person reflecting about the change taking place. In other words, experiencing something for the first time can make you feel strange and uncomfortable, or perhaps you are unsure about what is expected of you or what you can or should expect from yourself.

Stage 2 relates to you examining your use of knowledge and any potential gaps in your knowledge. Also, in stage 2, you would identify how the situation made you feel and, conversely, how you may have influenced the situation through your experience or inexperience. The purpose here is to connect feelings, knowledge and information with the situation and the individual so that the person can develop new insights.

Stage 3 clarifies what these insights are by describing them as 'outcomes of reflection' and how this learning will be taken forward (Atkins & Murphy, 1995, p. 2).

# Model of reflection from a student's perspective

Another model that you may find useful is the one developed by Stephenson and described in the chapter by Stephenson and Holm (1994) in the book by Palmer et al. (1994). This is based on students questioning their roles, feelings, actions, expectations and knowledge, as well as some of the broader surrounding issues within which their experiences may be embedded. These questions are extremely relevant to your stage of learning and are particularly helpful as they ask you to relate your professional practice to the wider political and social world, which may exert influence over what is happening and what you can do.

The main questions of Stephenson's model are as shown in the box.

## Concept summary: Stephenson's model of reflection (From a student's perspective)

- What was my role in the situation?
- Did I feel comfortable or uncomfortable? Why?
- What actions did I take?
- How did I and others act?
- Was it appropriate?
- How could I have improved the situation for myself, the patient, my practice supervisor?
- How can I change in future?
- Do I feel as if I have learnt anything new about myself?
- Did I expect anything different to happen? What and why?
- Has it changed my way of thinking in any way?

*(Continued)*

(Continued)

- What knowledge from theory and research can I apply to this situation?
- What broader issues, for example, political or social, arise from this situation?
- What do I think about these broader issues?

(*Source*: Stephenson, 1993, cited in Palmer et al., 1994)

The more experienced practitioner may want to use these questions with students as part of the teaching and assessing process to develop reflective learning together.

The penultimate model, offered by Howatson-Jones (2010), suggests exploratory questions that are meant to stimulate reflective thinking from a broader historical sense. These stem from personal research and are particularly relevant to reflections about working with people.

### Concept summary: A biographical perspective on reflection

- What foreknowledge did I bring to the situation and what do I need to know?
- What action did I take in the situation and why?
- How might others' perceptions be framing their responses?
- What is the quality of the response and how does it make me feel and act?
- What connections are there between responses now and earlier?
- Are there contraindications? Why?
- What, from autobiography, is influencing my noticing?
- What other factors might be influencing the situation?
- What does the language used in, or about, the situation reveal?
- What dimensions does my learning take, for example, psychological, physiological, affective (behavioural), spiritual or biographical?

(*Source*: Howatson-Jones, 2010)

The questions offered in the Howatson-Jones (2010) model provide an excellent opportunity to reflect on how your biography can be active in what you notice and how you might reflect. In Scenario 4.1, Jane brings her foreknowledge of other doctor–patient interactions to reflect on the differences in the consultant's communication. She also thinks about possible reasons for his different attitude based on her own autobiographical experience of having been a patient herself. This is an important point to question to ensure that blind spots do not develop, because these can hinder the ability to respond in better ways. Equally, developing biographical understanding can help you to read situations in different ways and understand why the consultant's approach might work better in one area than another.

The term 'model' is sometimes used interchangeably with the term 'reflective cycle'. Both offer structure to help you examine your reflective learning. Some, however, are more cyclical and are therefore referred to as reflective cycles. We now explore some reflective cycles.

# Reflective cycles

Reflective cycles offer the possibility to connect what has been learnt from one experience with what has been learnt from another. Using a reflective cycle can help you to clarify how learning is progressing and what you need to do to support it further, and it enables you to plan further action and set objectives relating to this. There are several different reflective cycles. One of the best-known reflective cycles is that of Gibbs (1988), which outlines specific steps to guide the learner through processes of description, acknowledgement of feelings, evaluation, analysis and action planning, as outlined in Figure 4.1.

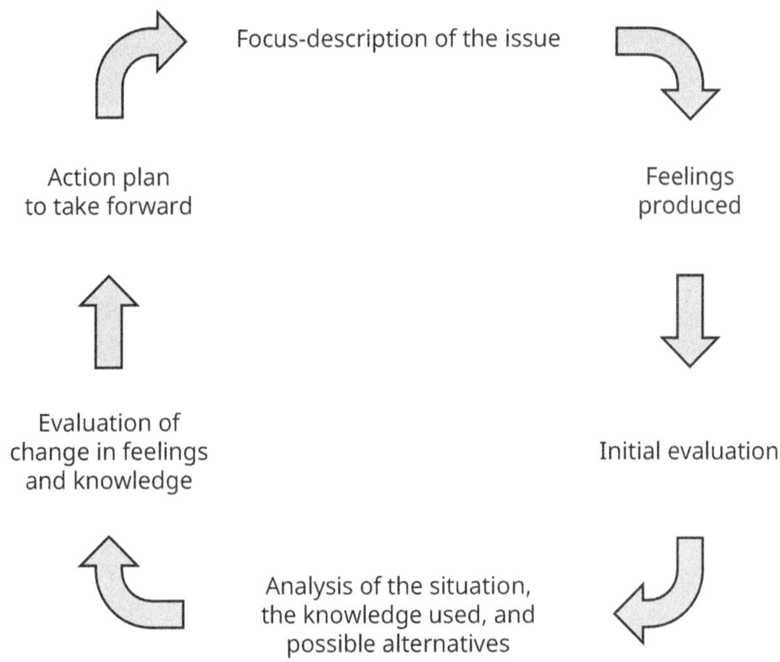


*Figure 4.1* Reflective cycle (adapted from Gibbs, 1988)

The description of the situation is limited to the salient points, which are the main priorities. By acknowledging feelings, the learner can consider processes, such as how to deal with sometimes difficult emotions that may be aroused by caring work and learning. Evaluation entails thinking about what the main issues are. These can then be analysed in greater detail by considering what knowledge is available, or might need to be developed, what other choices may have been accessible in the situation and the possible consequences if one of those choices had been selected instead. From this analysis follows consideration of changes to thinking about this type of situation, and how maybe to proceed the next time. From here, further action is then planned. The important aspects of this cycle are that analysis should result in some kind of action planning to take learning forward.

Now apply Gibbs' reflective cycle to Case Study 4.1 from the start of the chapter by completing Activity 4.4.

## Activity 4.4 Reflective cycle: Reflection

- Using the key stages of Gibbs' (1988) reflective cycle, identify which parts of Case Study 4.1 fit with these key stages. It may help to write these out on a separate piece of paper.
- Now underline the words within the parts of the example that represent the action points of the key stages of the reflective cycle under which you have placed them.

*There is an outline answer to this activity at the end of the chapter.*

From applying Gibbs' (1988) reflective cycle to Case Study 4.1, you may have identified that Jane needed to learn more about attentive listening to develop her own communication skills. A developed cycle based on Gibbs can be found in the Davis model, which includes an additional stage of considering the evidence base for change (Davis et al., 2011). You are directed to the book *Learning Skills for Nursing Students* (Davis et al., 2011), also in this series, to learn more. We proceed now to look at a different reflective cycle.

Driscoll's (2007, p. 44) reflective cycle has its roots in experiential learning and views reflection as a process of interrogating:

- What?
- So what?
- Now what?

These three questions encompass the need to be clear in the interpretation, interrogation and presentation of learning through reflection. The 'what?' refers to being able to describe the situation in words. This requires some mental ordering of events and helps to start the reflective process. In Case Study 4.1, Jane has started to build a therapeutic relationship with Sarah in the waiting room and then attends Sarah's consultation with her permission. She was surprised by the consultant's communication approach because it was different from what she had previously experienced. The 'so what?' involves beginning to analyse important aspects of the experience from which new discoveries may appear. When Jane starts to analyse what is important in this situation, she becomes aware that it is the quality of active listening, which the consultant demonstrated, that is different from other healthcare professional–patient interactions of which she has been part. The 'now what?' proposes new actions based on these discoveries, which may be reworked in multiple different situations. Jane realises that, in the past, she has not always been really focused on what people are saying to her and that this is a skill she needs to practise and use within her communication in the future. Driscoll's (2007) cycle is simple but effective. It is easy to remember, and these questions can easily be asked as part of most conversations within the classroom or practice and, therefore, can multiply the opportunities for reflection.

As suggested earlier, you may have noticed some similarities for the various frameworks, models and cycles of reflection. The next cycle acknowledges this point and is founded on the main principles we have looked at so far.

Jasper (2003, p. 2) suggests that most cycles of reflection are founded on the principles of experience–reflection–action (ERA). As with the previous examples, this reflective cycle starts with an experience or situation in which you are, or have been, involved. Experience may be something recent or something that you have developed. Reflection relates to reviewing and looking at the familiar, as well as the unfamiliar, with fresh eyes to consider what resources are available to you, who is, or needs to be, involved and what other strategies are available to you. Action refers to the implementation of learning and new strategies. These cycles of reflection may spiral from one to another over time (Jasper, 2003), forming part of a process of becoming as the person develops themselves and their knowledge (Johns, 2025). In other words, by connecting learning from different reflective episodes, you will be in a better position to get a clearer view of how you are developing your knowledge of yourself, your profession, your environment and your culture, and of other people, as well as the theoretical knowledge that underpins this. Reflection is about being able to connect experience with what you do.

The final model, specifically developed for those on a nursing preparation programme uses the basis of the familiar SBAR (Situation, Background, Assessment, and Recommendation) communication technique. This structure is used to convey information about those in our care quickly and was developed for the US Navy. The newly developed model considers the three stages of reflection: before action, in action and on action (Schon 1991; Edwards, 2017) and embeds these stages into the **C-Bar** (Horn & Jackson, 2025) framework to ensure that we cover all salient points and do not just merely describe any situation on which we wish to reflect. This is often where practitioners experience issues with the reflective process. The C-Bar model was explicitly developed for novice practitioners and those who have difficulty expressing feelings in written form or who are unable to describe them, a factor common in many reflective models (Bjerkvik & Hilli, 2019). Which is often where research indicates critically analysing is difficult for all levels of nurses at any career stage. The resolution stage of the C-Bar model aims to solve this for practitioners.

**C = Circumstances**

- Describe what happened/is happening.
- Who was present.
- Write down if there was/is anything you did not expect.

**B = Before**

- Did you think about what was happening before you acted.
- If so, describe what you thought about.
- What aspects of you gave you this knowledge? Was it an experience, life skills, or values or something else.

**A = Action**

- How did you respond to the situation?
- How did others respond to the situation?

**R = Resolution**

- What did you learn from this episode:

about yourself;

about others;

for your practice;

for your studies;

to share with others.

- What will you take forward with your practice?
- What would you do differently next time?
- What are the benefits for you personally and professionally on completing this reflection?

(Horn & Jackson, 2025)

An example of an autobiographical reflection written by Nancy from her personal life experience and reflected upon to enhance good nursing practice.

**C = Circumstances** I went to the optician with a friend, the technician asked how old we were because if we were 60, we'd get a discount as a thank you for "making it for so long". I was quite shocked that she viewed us both as old. I am not sure the technician realised that "making it for so long" made us feel they were ageist. I used humour to deflect my hurt.

**B = Before** I didn't really think too much before I responded as I was shocked. I thought the comment was ageist and this was the first time I have experienced this. I am aware of the Equality Act 2010 and have read extensively about pathological labelling within healthcare.

**A = Action** I was shocked. I am not sure how my friend felt as I did not ask her afterwards.

**R = Resolution**

I learnt and reconfirmed that I disagree with ageism towards any age group in society, and that others do not have the same ethos. This episode has strengthened my resolve to see the person and not their age and to treat everyone kindly. Next time I may be more direct when a virtual stranger comments in this way. I would also have a reflective discussion with my friend based on what I was thinking to compare our experiences of this and to check she was okay, and to seek a different resolution/viewpoint. By doing all of this I would be enhancing my reflective skills, which would improve nursing practice and my personal life.

Having looked at several reflective frameworks, models and cycles, now complete Activity 4.5 to clarify your understanding of them.

## Activity 4.5 Critical thinking

- What are the main commonalities and differences for the various frameworks, models, and cycles?
- Which of them appear easier to use and why?
- Which of them appear harder to use and why?
- Are there different types of situations that the different frameworks, models, and cycles are suited to? If so, why?
- What do you see as the strengths and limitations of each of the frameworks, models and cycles?

*There is an outline answer to this activity at the end of the chapter.*

## Chapter summary

This chapter has introduced and explored several different reflective frameworks, models and cycles that you can choose from when starting or continuing to reflect.

Through the case studies and activities, you can apply a variety of reflective formats. These give you a starting point from which to develop your own reflective journey. Nevertheless, they assist with structuring what might sometimes be painful and difficult to admit to yourself, as well as help you to identify how to replicate and multiply successes. When time is short, the discipline of a reflective framework can help keep you on track. How to create space for such reflection is explored in greater depth in the next chapter.

## Brief outline answers

In this section, answers to the chapter's activities will be outlined and explained.

### Activity 4.2 Evidence-based practice and reflection

You may have observed that your practice supervisor, lecturer, or advanced practitioner could talk around the subject effortlessly while undertaking the tasks of practice or teaching. For example, perhaps your practice supervisor was adjusting a wound dressing in response to the nonverbal cues of your patient, whilst telling them what the wound dressing was for and how the wound healing was progressing. Similarly, in a clinical science class you may have observed the lecturer responding to some students' confusion by asking class members to take on the role of oxygen and sit in a haemoglobin 'car' made up of four chairs that could take four passengers. Maybe you observed an advanced practitioner skilfully completing an examination while teaching the patient and you. There might have been a fleeting hesitation while the practice supervisor, lecturer or advanced practitioner took in the cues they received from the patient/class, but the alteration in what they did next would have been imperceptible. However, if the patient asks a question of the practice supervisor or a student asks the lecturer, there is a more perceptible pause to think of the answer to give. The answer is likely to have involved some dialogue to check whether it met the expectation of the questioner and that they also understood the answer.

### Activity 4.3 Critical thinking

You may have considered issues relating to developing pressure ulcers. You and your practice supervisor or your student may have noted a change in skin colour and appearance. There may have been a difference in interpreting the severity of the problem due to different knowledge levels. You may not have realised this until comparing the scores you took, and you may have discovered that, when using some scoring systems, it is easy to overestimate risk. You may have been surprised by the degree of subjectivity involved. If you are an experienced practitioner, you may have considered your accountability if the patient were to develop a pressure ulcer. You may have been more careful to assess the risk regularly using the same tool each time to monitor changes. You may have learnt that assessment tools are only as good as the knowledge and observation of the person using them. In your reflection, try to relate your scenario to *The Code* (NMC, 2018b), for example, *Practise effectively* (items 10.2 and 10.3) and *Preserve safety* (items 13.1 and 13.2).

As suggested in Case Study 4.1, in Activity 4.1 and again in this activity, much of our learning occurs through experience. This is often an unconscious process, which, as a professional engaged in life-long learning, we need to make more of a conscious process. This is where the activities of reflection-in-action and reflection-on-action become important. This process can, however, be difficult to unpick and it might be interesting to read Patricia Benner's (1984) influential work in which she discusses the process 'from novice to expert' in terms of learning. It is good to be mindful that one of Benner's key premises is that, as we develop, we tend to 'read' situations in context rather than in isolation. It may then be beneficial to you, when discussing something you have seen a colleague do (this could be your practice supervisor, your student or another healthcare professional), to try to reduce the activity to smaller steps, in order to discuss the underlying decision-making associated with each step and how this information informed their next step.

### Activity 4.4 Reflective cycle: Reflection

Answers to this activity will be broken down into description, feelings, evaluation, analysis, evaluation of change, and action planning.

## Description

Jane was working in an outpatient department in the second year of her nurse apprentice programme. The consultant examined Sarah and listened to her concerns and then explained further processes. He allowed Sarah time to develop further questions.

## Feelings

Jane was surprised by the empathetic communication style used by the consultant.

## Evaluation

Jane noted that the consultant had attended to what Sarah was saying and how Sarah was processing the information he gave her. Jane wondered why the consultant behaved so differently to her previous experience of such consultations.

## Analysis

Retrospectively, Jane wondered whether the consultant had been a patient at some point and been frustrated at the way people communicated with him. Perhaps a family member or friend had been the patient, and he had tried to support them. She considered how different the consultant had been in the way he had attended to what Sarah was saying, and to her body language revealing she was feeling overwhelmed, and how the consultant had allowed Sarah time to absorb what he was being told and gain the answers to her questions. Jane thought about the impact the consultant's communication style had on making Sarah feel listened to, and the positive working atmosphere of the team. She identified that what she saw was an effective working culture in action. In reflecting on this scenario, it is recommended that you refer to *The Code* (NMC, 2018b); for example, *Prioritise people* (items 1.1, 1.5 and 2.6) and *Practise effectively* (items 8.3 and 8.6).

## Evaluation of change

Jane thought about how she could develop her own active listening skills to enhance her practice.

## Action planning

Jane would read more about communication, particularly in relation to active and attentive listening, and she would continue to reflect on her experiences and keep a reflective log of her progress to discuss with her practice supervisor.

## Activity 4.5 Critical thinking

The autobiographical reflection is a personal piece and no answers are incorrect

- You may have identified that the areas of commonality between the different reflective formats include evaluation, analysis and action. Areas of difference might be in the depth of reflection demanded by the models compared with the easier application of the reflective cycles. The biographical model is also different in asking you to take note and identify what you are consciously noticing.
- Perhaps reflection-in-action was particularly relevant in starting to develop your practice skills, whereas reflection-on-action may have helped you to embed them. The reflective cycles, perhaps, helped you structure reflection within assignments and when talking about practice. The models of reflection may have helped to examine your learning in more detail through reflective writing.
- You may have noticed problem-solving as a strength of reflection-in-action, whereas insufficient consciousness of the learning achieved may have been a limitation. Similarly, too much thought may be a barrier to developing reflection-on-action during activities. A strength of reflective models could be the potential depth for reflection they offer, but the time needed for this could be a limitation. Perhaps you viewed the acknowledgement of feelings in some of the models and reflective cycles as a strength that helps to take feelings forward in more positive ways, but the simplicity of the reflective cycles may also encourage superficial examination of issues. Conceivably, the biographical approach helped you to integrate your

reflective learning better, but this may also have been challenging in what you found out about yourself. You may also have wondered about the importance of credible evidence on which to base changing practice.

## Further reading

**Ellis, P.** (2026). *Evidence-based practice in nursing* (6th ed.). Sage/Learning Matters.

This book incorporates reflective dispositions of the nurse within a model of evidence-based practice in nursing.

**Gibbs, G.** (1988). *Learning by doing: A guide to teaching and learning methods.* Oxford Polytechnic, Further Education Unit.

**Johns, C.** (2025). *Becoming a reflective practitioner* (7th ed.). John Wiley.

**Moon, J.** (2013). *Reflection in learning and professional development: Theory and practice.* Taylor & Francis.

**Taylor, B.** (2010). *Reflective practice for healthcare professionals* (3rd ed.). Open University Press.

These books offer in-depth explanations of some of the models and frameworks discussed in this chapter.

## Useful websites

**https://www.nmc.org.uk/globalassets/sitedocuments/standards/supporting-information-for-reflection-in-nursing-and-midwifery-practice.pdf**

A useful document from the NMC outlining ways of learning from practice.

**https://reflection.ed.ac.uk/reflectors-toolkit**

This resource from the University of Edinburgh has useful tips for successful reflective practice.

# Chapter 5 Creating space for reflection

## NMC Future Nurse: Standards of Proficiency for Registered Nurses

This chapter will address the following platforms and proficiencies:

**Platform 5: Leading and managing nursing care and working in teams**

5.9 Demonstrate the ability to challenge and provide constructive feedback about care delivered by others in the team and support them to identify and agree individual learning needs.

**Platform 6: Improving safety and quality of care**

6.9 Work with people, their families, carers, and colleagues to develop effective improvement strategies for quality and safety, sharing feedback and learning from positive outcomes and experiences, mistakes and adverse outcomes and experiences.

6.11 Acknowledge the need to accept and manage uncertainty and demonstrate an understanding of strategies that develop resilience in self and others.

## Chapter aims

After reading this chapter you will be able to:

- define the concept of transitional space;
- identify some barriers and limitations to reflection and strategies for overcoming these;
- examine the kinds of relationships that exist between people and how these might be more caring and compassionate;
- consider how you negotiate your position within healthcare;
- identify what makes spaces compelling for reflection and learning.

## Case Study 5.1: George

George had worked for some years as a registered nurse on a neurological ward where he had nursed Ms Gillespie. Ms Gillespie had, at that time, been newly diagnosed with a brain tumour and was admitted for investigations and to stabilise her with medication. At first Ms Gillespie was highly emotional and confided in George that, as she, too, had been a nurse and knew what was in store for her, she did not want to live with any disability or burden her long-time partner. Sometime later, Ms Gillespie was admitted again with severe hemiplegia, hemianopia and dysphagia. She recognised George and became quite tearful on seeing him. George was surprised and relieved to see that Ms Gillespie indicated that she was content and seemed to have found a level of acceptance of her condition and they could still laugh together.

A few years later George was working night duty with the community palliative care team and was allocated a client whose name was familiar. When he arrived at the address, he instantly recognised Ms Gillespie, who had been assigned care as she was nearing the end of her life. Ms Gillespie recognised George, and he could see she was pleased to see him. Ms Gillespie's partner, Ms Tucker, seemed weary and non-communicative; George could only imagine that the years and strain of Ms Gillespie's illness had impacted on her and on their relationship. George at the end of his final shift with Ms Gillespie, she took his hand and, tearfully, told him that they would not see each other again because she felt sure that she would die before the day was out. Going home, George felt sad at leaving Ms Gillespie for a final time because they had developed a bond over the years. That evening, George was called by the palliative care team's coordinator to say that Ms Gillespie had, indeed, died that afternoon.

## Activity 5.1 Reflection

Think about Case Study 5.1: you may find that questions arise for you. For example, what do you think of the way in which Ms Gillespie seemed to reset her boundaries as her illness progressed? What could the potential challenges be in supporting her and her partner, Ms Tucker? Try to put yourself in George's position: what would you be thinking about this situation?

Make a note of where/when you think you could have the most beneficial reflection.

This is your own reflection, but an outline answer has been included at the end of the chapter.

# Introduction

Case Study 5.1 illustrates how we are sometimes confronted by situations where people's reactions can resonate with emotions and/or uncertainties we are experiencing. Finding the time or a suitable place for reflection is difficult as it is often easy to prioritise other things, perhaps because reflection reveals things that make us uncomfortable. It is easy to 'ignore' these feelings but continuing with familiar and comfortable ways of thinking and doing things keeps us from exploring alternatives and considering change. Transition means moving from one position, or point of view to another and this shift between positions can feel uncomfortable and uncertain. As you progress through your nursing programme and your career, more is expected from you in terms of knowledge, skills, and decision-making.

This chapter introduces the concept of reflection as a **transitional space** in which you are encouraged to explore, develop and grow. The chapter considers some of the barriers and limitations to reflection and strategies you can use to overcome these. Chapter 5 asks you to examine relationships that exist between individuals, and how you negotiate your place in diverse healthcare situations. Finally, the chapter explores care and compassion for yourself and others, and what makes spaces compelling for reflection and learning.

# Finding the time and space for reflection

Finding the time and space for reflection requires interest, motivation, and commitment, as discussed in previous chapters. Taylor (2010) suggests that reflection should be undertaken daily and making reflection part of your routine means that you are more likely to continue with it and be able to see trends and changes taking place in both your practice and learning. This view suggests that, just as in Activity 5.1, space for reflection can be found at some point in the day. However, spaces for reflection frequently appear at the margins of activity and are necessarily often brief and hurried.

While in Chapter 9, we discuss reflective writing in more detail, at this point it is pertinent to add that theorists such as Dewey, Kolb, Schön and Johns all discuss reflection as something we should internalise, meaning that it can occur at any time and as a more or less continual process. Stevens and Cooper (2009) discuss this in some detail, highlighting Dewey's (1933) idea of developing a *habit of thinking in a reflective way*. Similarly, Kolb (1984) and Schön (2009) discuss learning from experience, a key source in developing professional attitude, dexterity and critical thinking in nursing. Johns (2025) takes this idea further and suggests that being a reflective practitioner is a 'way of being' and follows on from practising reflection and understanding ourselves. With this in mind, please consider Case Study 5.2 to help you identify where such spaces might appear in both personal and professional life.

## Case Study 5.2: After hours with George

After leaving Ms Gillespie, George cycled home, showered, had breakfast and went to bed to sleep for the day. Sleeping was fitful, so when the phone rang at 18.30 and it was the palliative care team's coordinator to say that Ms Gillespie had died at 16.00, it was not a shock for George – somehow, he had expected it. George called his friends to meet them at a bar later and went for an hour's run along the beach. The bar with friends was great fun as it turned out to be karaoke evening and everyone was keen to have a turn with the microphone. It was late to bed for George that night.

## Activity 5.2 Reflection

- Which activities could have offered George opportunities for reflection?
- Write down how you manage with situations that you find distressing.
- What strategies do you use to reach closure?

*There is an outline answer to this question at the end of the chapter.*

Through this case study you may have identified that there is scope and space for reflection. It is, however, your focus, willingness, and commitment to reflect that are necessary to maximise your learning. When time is limited, other priorities take over and it becomes difficult to maintain the discipline required for reflecting on learning in different situations both inside and outside the classroom and in practice.

One way to maintain reflection is to use supportive mechanisms, such as reflecting with others, either in groups or by choosing a critical friend, who can invite commitment and provide additional support (Bulman & Schutz, 2013). Such support makes it easier to face and deal with the changes that reflection inevitably brings. Peer support is important to reflection in that it offers the opportunity for a two-way process of learning from dialogue (Johns, 2025). Such dialogue involves reflective telling as well as reflective receiving. For example, when discussing how you feel with someone, they are likely to ask you what sparked that emotion, which will stimulate you to reflect on some of the surrounding reasons and issues. Equally, your listener may then think about your reasoning and offer their own experiences after reflecting on what you have said. In this way, reflection is mutually beneficial. In Case Study 5.1, the transition being experienced by Ms Gillespie and her partner resonated with George's uncertainties of emotional boundaries as a nurse. The reflective questioning in George's example was primarily internal and it may have been helpful for George to share his thoughts with a colleague or, in the case of a student nurse, with their practice supervisor.

As nurses, it is important to recognise that practice is complex, constantly evolving and full of surprises. This means that it is essential for self-reflection to be a part of everyday practice. Therefore, peer-reflective dialogue needs to be recognised as a normal part of professional practice. Although we might realise the importance of peer-reflective dialogue from a theoretical perspective, we often do not take the time to initiate or engage with colleagues to discuss our experiences (Sundgren, 2021). We might think that this moment of contemplation is only necessary for the inexperienced, but nothing could be further from the truth. Let us consider the kind of space created by reflection.

## Transitional space

Transitional space is, as the name suggests, a place where we are in the process of change. Jarvis (2006) identifies that learning means that people move from a position of 'being' to one of 'becoming'. This means that, in the process of adjustment, a person enters a transitional space where there are possibilities for development and where they become changed as people. This learning is not coincidental but needs to be negotiated and to do this requires self-awareness and self-knowledge and a discussion with a practice supervisor, lecturer or colleague. For example, you probably entered your nursing programme with an understanding of who you were but, as the programme progressed, this understanding may have shifted as you 'became' a nurse. Similarly, if you are an experienced practitioner, you have an idea of the kind of practitioner you are. Nevertheless, as you gather experience you become more expert, perhaps as a manager, a nurse specialist, an advanced practitioner or a nurse educator.

### Activity 5.3 Reflection

Now consider your development since starting the programme or, if you are a registered nurse, your development in the past few years.

Make a note of if, when and how you negotiated this learning.

Could you have made more use of situations to learn?

Were you proactive in your learning?

How could you do things differently if you were able to turn back the clock?

*As this is a personal reflection, there is no outline answer to this activity.*

Transitional space, originally conceptualised by Winnicott (1965), is also defined as the point where subjective inner experience interacts with objective outer experience (Andrew et al., 2009; Hunt & West, 2007). For example, George was faced with an emotive situation in which Ms Gillespie shared awareness of her transition. For George, each contact with Ms Gillespie over the years, and in their final moment of farewell, meant that he was also experiencing transition:

- in his relationship with the service user;
- in needing to realign his emotionality with the external cues provided by Ms Gillespie and her partner;
- by learning to deal with his own emotions and 'reinterpret' them in terms of what he interpreted as 'professional behaviour'.

The transitional space of learning is framed by how organisations and individuals:

- help to create such a space;
- perceive themselves;
- interact.

The following case study provides an example to illustrate these processes.

### Case Study 5.3: Ellen's experience of failure

Ellen was at the end of the first year of her nurse apprentice programme and had recently received results that required her to retake the clinical science examination. The classes had been difficult to concentrate on, and Ellen acknowledged that she did not like the subject.

Ellen was disappointed because she had worked hard and felt there was limited feedback as to where she had gone wrong. Her initial thought was that expectations of the apprentice were unfair, and she felt upset with her tutor who, Ellen felt, had not explained things clearly. Ellen was tempted to leave the programme because this felt so insurmountable. As her initial upset subsided, she started considering what she could do. Her friend Mitch had passed the exam and encouraged Ellen to take the second attempt and offered to help with her revision.

During revision, Ellen realised that she had focused on a few body systems in too much depth but had not revised the module learning outcomes. Her knowledge of the systems she had covered was good and she started to feel more in control and confident. Ellen learnt that her study technique needed adjusting and, by focusing on the module learning outcomes, she felt confident of passing the examination. In all, Ellen had learnt a valuable lesson; namely, how to manage disappointment and keep going; she had become more resilient when confronted by adversity.

These case studies demonstrate that transitional space is a place where we learn and develop from situations by reviewing the interaction between:

- our subjective experience and
- the feedback from the external world; namely the people we interact with and manage circumstances we find ourselves in.

Activity 5.4 helps you identify where transitional space might be within your own life and how you are learning and changing.

### Activity 5.4 Reflection

Activity 5.4 has two elements to it. Firstly, think of a time of significant change or learning in your life and answer the following questions:

- What were the circumstances?
- What were you thinking at the time?
- What did you learn?
- What change was brought about?
- Have you changed as a person as a result of the event?
- How did what you learned influence the change?
- Have you noticed any further changes; when and where have these occurred?

*There is an outline answer to this activity at the end of the chapter.*

For the second part of this learning activity, choose and write down information about a situation in which you met unexpected challenges or changes in practice. An example of this might be to reflect on a situation that occurred during a very busy time, such as working in an unfamiliar setting, using extensive personal protective equipment (PPE) or having to care for extremely ill and dying patients, such as during the COVID-19 pandemic. Now answer the same list of questions as in the first part of this learning activity and write down your answers, as you will return to this in Activity 5.5. Next consider any similarities and differences between the first and second parts of this learning activity.

As the second part of this activity is based on a specific personal situation there is no outline answer at the end of the chapter.

The first part of Activity 5.4 may have focused on personal circumstances, such as:

- how you developed as a person before and/or during your nursing programme (and after it if you are an experienced practitioner);
- on learning.

The second part is focused on learning through experience in your professional capacity. In both activities you may recognise that learning from those around us places us in a transitional space because we are challenged to adjust our subjective meaning of what is being asked. By identifying where transitional spaces have appeared in your life, you can consider which barriers and limitations impact on your ability to reflect and learn.

## Barriers and limitations to reflection

Although reflection offers opportunities for us to develop our learning, it may be inhibited by certain challenges. Some of the difficulties that may create barriers to reflection include:

- not knowing how to reflect: you get stuck with how things feel and cannot make sense of things;
- tiredness: too much effort is required to maintain mental focus;
- lack of time: life gets in the way;
- not realising that reflection and learning can occur subconsciously and may result in the reinforcement of 'negative' ideas;
- lack of insight: it is difficult to recognise how personal actions might affect others;
- distractions: it is difficult to find a quiet space;
- lack of motivation: you cannot see the relevance of reflection;
- finding it difficult to manage the consequences of reflection: reflection is too painful or revealing.

When we engage in reflection, different factors could limit the learning we accomplish. According to Smith and Jack (2005), these factors constitute the following:

- Some learning styles help you engage with reflection more readily and in more meaningful ways than others.
- It is not always easy for practitioners to articulate the knowledge they have, and you may not always be able to discern your supervisor's decision-making thoughts and process.
- You may not have evidence-based up-to-date knowledge.
- Reflection may be used for instrumental purposes and discontinued; in other words, reflection may remain focused on a course requirement, limiting you to a specific way of thinking.

Several of these factors relate to personal understanding of what reflection is and what your role is within the process, with some being remedied by deepening your knowledge of reflection. We can overcome other factors, such as taking time and space for reflection, but it takes effort and motivation to create the necessary space. Taking steps to overcome the barriers should come from recognising this as an opportunity to design our own learning. Limitations to reflection often result in the depth of reflection we achieve and engaging in a reflective cycle without fully analysing what is happening and why; it results in limited learning due to the reflection being superficial or unconscious (Loughran, 2002).

An alternative to overcoming these barriers and limitations is to ask a colleague or practice supervisor to help you with reflective processing. This means being able to share your thinking with someone else in a way that challenges your thinking as something that is developing, as illustrated in Case Study 5.1. This could expose elements of your 'becoming' to others, but it is an important part of demonstrating progression and articulating how you are applying your knowledge in different situations. The next section considers how you might do this in diverse healthcare settings.

# Negotiating your place in diverse healthcare settings

A key aspect of 'becoming' is through negotiating your position in different settings and developing the professional self (Barchard, 2022). This occurs through developing your role and idea of who you are and who you need to be in different arenas. For example, the role of the nurse in an emergency department (ED) will be quite different from working in mental health, paediatric, learning disability or community settings. In the ED, the nurse's role focuses on rapid problem-solving, whereas in other settings the nurse will be working collaboratively with the people in their care and problem-solving may have a longer timescale. Although you would be caring and empathetic in all situations, you may need to be more assertive in the ED, and this could result in a different development. To negotiate your position within a particular setting, you need to understand your role in relation to your stage of preparation and the nurse's role within the multiprofessional healthcare team. This involves:

- preparing to enter the new setting: understanding key care priorities of the setting and identifying potential learning opportunities;
- being aware of ongoing changes and embracing these and the opportunities they offer;
- reflecting on your current knowledge: mapping your knowledge to that of the care priorities of the setting and planning to address any deficits, possibly through drafting a **learning contract**;
- reflecting on what you are doing, the feedback you get and how you see yourself developing, while in that care setting;
- summarising what you have learnt about the care setting and yourself;
- reflecting on how any knowledge you have gained might be applicable in different settings.

Preparing, reflecting and summarising are important features to help us make sense of how we develop meaning from different activities and settings. Activity 5.5 allows you to apply and think about some of these issues, to learn from your experiences.

## Activity 5.5 Reflection

This learning activity consists of two parts. Firstly, consider the different placements you have had (or if you are an experienced practitioner, the different positions you have held). How did you:

- prepare for the placement or role?
- experience change?
- identify others' expectations of you?
- understand your position in the setting?

*(Continued)*

(Continued)

- develop your learning in the setting?
- develop your identity?
- feel when you left the setting and why did you feel that way?
- plan what to do next?

For the second part, answer the same questions in relation to the scenario that you chose for the second part of Activity 5.4. Write down your answers. Now consider any similarities and differences between the first and second parts of this learning activity.

*As this activity is based on your own experiences, there is no outline answer at the end of the chapter.*

Perhaps you prepared differently for a planned change of work environment or an unexpected change. Maybe you had to manage personal anxieties and perceived dangers; if so, how did you cope and did this impact on your quality of care? You may have left one setting with a more positive feeling than another. Working through how you prepared to enter the setting, reflecting on what you learnt and your developing identity while you were there, you can connect the past with the present and a potential future. Discussing these issues with your practice supervisor or colleague is an important aspect of negotiating a transitional space for learning as it allows you to understand and identify areas of past, current and future development.

Another aspect of negotiating your position relates to the levels of dependence, independence and interdependence that you may adopt or be allowed to take on. When negotiating our position, previous experiences (as highlighted in Chapter 3) influence our perceptions of others and ourselves (Andrew et al., 2009; Hunt & West, 2007). This could result in projecting the role of parent on to the supervisor, which can distort some of our responses. This process is illustrated within Case Study 5.4.

## Case Study 5.4: Ravi's experience of two practice supervisors

Ravi, a third-year mental health nurse, allocated to a specialised crisis intervention team. He had just returned to complete his mandatory placement time which he had lost due to sickness. Ravi also needed to continue to be assessed to complete his practice assessment. His practice assessor, Sylvia, had been critical of his performance during the initial placement and he now felt apprehensive as she had asked to have a formal meeting with him.

During their discussion, Sylvia told Ravi he was not meeting his practice assessment objectives. Going through them together she identified that Ravi needed constant guidance, he was waiting to be told what to do rather than working proactively. At this stage Sylvia expected him to give input into the care planning discussions with those in the care of the team. Highlighting that Ravi should be making suggestions independently, without being prompted by herself or other registered nurses in the team. She showed concern as to whether Ravi would pass the practice assessment and told him he needed to become more proactive in his interactions with the people in his care and staff to do so.

Ravi explained that he knew what to do but needed confirmation that this was correct. After the meeting, Ravi was demoralised, unsure how he could improve and felt that everything he did was wrong. Ravi was due to work with another supervisor for the next two weeks as Sylvia was on leave.

Ravi met with his new supervisor, Wendy, on Monday the following week. Wendy when working with Ravi facilitated discussions and Ravi's confidence grew during the first week. He began to think that he would pass this assessment because Wendy told him he was working more independently and meeting the objectives that first week. On the last week of his placement Sylvia returned, although there were a few areas for development, both Sylvia and Wendy were satisfied that Ravi had passed his practice assessment.

## Activity 5.6 Reflection

- In what ways were Ravi's initial behaviour and responses unhelpful to his progression on placement?
- What else could he have done to help in negotiating his position?
- Access the following article to help you with the above.
- Trueland, J. (2022) Supervision and keeping the relationship positive, *Nursing Standard, 37*(6), pp. 24–26. *There are outline answers to these questions at the end of the chapter.*

As is noted in this case study, the quality of interactions can have a marked effect on our responses and ability to learn. When we are treated in what seem to be negative ways, we may often respond less confidently.

## Activity 5.7 Reflection

Now look back at your reflections in the second part of Activities 5.4 and 5.5.

- On reflection, how was your perception of the new environment influenced by your practice supervisor or staff members who were familiar with that clinical area?
- What was your role in negotiating a safe and supportive learning and work environment?

*As this activity is based on a specific personal situation there is no outline answer at the end of the chapter.*

Creating spaces for reflection includes using care and compassion to create a meaningful space for learning. Let us consider issues relating to care and compassion within spaces of reflection.

# Care and compassion

Care and compassion in terms of learning relate to how cared for you feel. Although the 6 Cs were developed for nurses caring for patients, we should also extend these to how we interact with each other. Nursing practice is sometimes so hectic that we barely have time to think, so we feel under constant pressure. Creating space for reflection is a form of self-care that allows us to review what is happening and take every opportunity to learn, enabling us to reach a different view of ourselves (Schmidt, 2008). Equally important, when creating space for self-care is practicing self-compassion, a vital part of the reflective process. This positive behaviour assists nurses at all levels to develop and demonstrate compassion for the self. Compassion is developed further and then demonstrated to those in the care of those who actively practice self-compassion. Kotera et al. (2021) tell us that there are three stages of self-compassion:

i being kind and understanding towards oneself (self-kindness),
ii acknowledging that suffering is part of human life (common humanity),
iii being present in the here and now (mindfulness).

As discussed in Chapter 3, biographical construction and reflection have the potential to change impressions and develop your learning in affirming ways that are compassionate. The ability to explore 'self' is an important element of self-caring (Chan & Schwind, 2006; Kotera et al., 2021). Activity 5.8 can help you to read situations differently and identify opportunities to become self-caring.

## Activity 5.8 Critical thinking

Look again at the case studies of Ellen's failure and Ravi's experience, and consider the following:

- Who showed care and compassion?
- How were care and compassion demonstrated, if at all?
- Were either Ellen or Ravi self-compassionate? If so, when?
- What were the results for Ellen and Ravi?
- What did they take forward from their situations?
- If care and compassion are absent, what is, or is likely to be, the outcome?
- How can we show self-care, self-compassion, care and compassion for others as a part of reflection?

When you have completed answering the above points, write a reflective summary of what you have learnt using the pro forma from Chapter 1, and include an action plan for how you can show care and compassion. Use this action plan to work towards the goals you have set yourself and reflect on your learning as you progress.

*There are outline answers to this activity at the end of the chapter.*

By working through Activity 5.8, you may have viewed the situations in more positive or affirmative ways. Reading situations from a more positive perspective can help to open a space that is more conducive to learning, not coercively, but by being open-minded and engaged. Now we will consider space for reflection and learning, which draws all the parts already discussed into a whole.

# Space that is compelling for reflection and learning

Space might be described as a **compelling space** (Horowitz, 2018), where people initiate opportunities by engaging with each other to learn something new. Such acts of initiation may relate to choosing:

- whether or not you reflect and learn;
- which design you use in your reflection.

In other words, do you choose to reflect with others, in written form or by thinking things through on your own? A compelling space is one that stimulates and invites meaningful learning and where people feel able to acknowledge that they do not know (Howatson-Jones, 2010). In such a space you are empowered to become proactive and develop curiosity, enquiry and meaning. Here, you have autonomy as to how you develop your own knowledge and take control of your learning. To do this you need to integrate the personal with the professional, as outlined in Chapter 3, and, in so doing, create a compelling space. In Case Study 5.1 George recognises his autonomy by allowing himself to reflect on his relationship with Ms Gillespie and how the situation impacts on his way of being. This illustrates how we can take more control of our own transitions to become a qualified nurse or within the context of life-long learning. The following Case Study offers an example of how a compelling space is created.

## Case Study 5.5: Jared's experience of a compelling space

Jared has been allocated to the ambulatory cancer care centre for the final placement of the adult nursing programme. Jared is enjoying this placement because there is no hierarchical distinction between the medical and nursing staff. They all work as a team in a person-centred way. A poem written by one of the patients was displayed in the waiting area and seemed to sum up these impressions for Jared.

*(Continued)*

(Continued)

Jared looked at the poem every day when arriving on duty and found inspiration for the day. This week, on finishing placement, Abby, Jared's practice supervisor, asked him to share some reflection and learning with the team. Jared began with the poem and told them all how he was inspired by the person-centred attitude of the team, and how learning had really developed in this area. The team gave positive feedback. Jared left placement feeling affirmed and valued. In his reflective diary Jared thought about what had helped his learning. It was a combination of the positive atmosphere, the team working together, the inspiration of the poem that motivated him and the team's feedback on his practice. All these elements made the space compelling for learning.

## Chapter summary

This chapter introduced the concept of transitional space, and the activities offer opportunities to examine transitional spaces in your own life. Barriers and limitations to reflection are addressed and include suggestions to overcome these to increase your reflective opportunities. The chapter examined how you negotiate your place within diverse healthcare settings and raise issues of care and compassion that influence the quality of the learning experience. Compelling spaces for learning and reflection are created through empowering individuals and Chapter 6 continues this theme by looking at reflection and reflexivity.

# Brief outline answers

In this section, answers to the chapter's activities will be outlined and explained.

### Activity 5.1 Reflection

You may have identified the following places/times for reflection:

- while making breakfast – contemplating your current knowledge base in a new setting;
- while relaxing – consider what information you want/need to find out;
- while exercising – combining physical and mental activity by revisiting new knowledge while doing repetitive exercises;
- while out with friends – through being in the midst of life and fun you would be placing life and death in perspective and realising that, as a nurse and even though you have an affection for those in your care, you cannot carry the whole world on your shoulders.

You may not have taken up these opportunities for reflection because of a lack of time, because you wanted to do something else or because you were tired; however, these suggestions could help you to combine everyday activities with reflective moments.

## Activity 5.2 Reflection

You may have considered the following activities as offering scope for reflection:

- undertaking systematic reflection using a recognised model, as discussed in Chapter 4;
- talking about practice with others: reflecting on observed practice and how this compared with knowledge;
- talking about the day with others: identifying your thoughts and highlighting positives and areas for further reflection;
- working with an expert/specialist: reflecting on differences between settings.

## Activity 5.4 Reflection

In considering the question about significant change in your life, you may have thought about when you were an adolescent, or maybe when you became a parent for the first time. Some of the feelings evoked are likely to have been anxiety and uncertainty. You may have learnt new skills and this in turn may have helped you to grow in confidence. You are likely to have become increasingly independent and able to make decisions for yourself. Modifications to these changes are likely to have ensued from problems you encountered and successes you experienced, so that there will have been further uncertain times, but also greater ability to direct your progression.

## Activity 5.6 Reflection

Ravi's previous experience on the ward with Sylvia had been anxiety provoking because of the way he perceived her constant criticism of him. Subconsciously, he was adopting a child's role of waiting to be told what to do, not to make mistakes. He perceived Sylvia in a parent's role of knowing best. With Wendy, Ravi was able to move to an adult role, recognising that he had space to give input and make decisions, but that Wendy was available if he encountered anything he did not understand or if he was uncertain. This situation should be recognisable; as student or qualified healthcare professional we will always encounter people who trigger this kind of response. Ravi should have spoken to Sylvia about their working relationship and negotiated how they could move forward. This might be difficult to do but it shows the characteristics of a professional; it takes courage and commitment (two of the 6 Cs) to address a situation where you feel vulnerable. If he felt unsure, Ravi should have spoken to his practice education facilitator or university link lecturer about his experiences as a way of helping him to negotiate his position and prepare for the return meeting, as they could have been present to support him as a student. In so doing, this could have created a learning situation for himself and Sylvia – a situation in which he could ask them both for feedback on his communication and interaction strategies. This would have been appropriate and proactive for Ravi as a final-year student nurse.

In your reflections on the second parts of Activities 5.4 and 5.5, you may have recognised the tensions that Ravi encountered. Consider how you responded to expectations in your new work environment. It is also worthwhile considering whether you discussed how you felt or your needs. Naturally, we should remain mindful that managing difficult or sensitive issues takes practice and confidence. It is, therefore, wise to start practising from the beginning of your programme so that, by the time you reach year 3, you will have built the necessary confidence and techniques. In this regard, read the section *Practise efficiently: Work cooperatively* of *The Code* (NMC, 2018b), which deals with appropriate referral of care to colleagues, and inter- and intraprofessional communication to ensure safety and quality of care (items 8.1–8.6).

## Activity 5.8 Critical thinking

Your answers may have included the following.

- Mitch showed care and compassion towards Ellen in the case study by helping her to revise, and Wendy showed care and compassion in working with Ravi by supervising at key points to ensure that he was not undermined but supported.
- Ellen adjusted her study and revision techniques, and Ravi functioned more independently.

- Ellen become more resilient to adversity and Ravi saw himself as a capable practitioner.
- Both Ellen and Ravi showed self-compassion by using ***reflection -on-action*** *after* each of the circumstances they found themselves in. They reflected by thinking about future strategies for improvement.
- Without care and compassion, people feel insecure and less capable and are more likely to make mistakes.
- Showing ourselves care and compassion involves getting to know ourselves better through some of the techniques suggested in this book. Showing care and compassion for others involves looking for positives rather than being negatively critical.

## Further reading

**Knud Illeris, K.** (2018). *Contemporary theories of learning: Learning theorists in their own words* (2nd ed.). Routledge.

This book offers an interesting overview of contemporary learning theories.

**Kotera, Y. et al.** (2021). Predicting self-compassion in UK nursing students: Relationships with resilience, engagement, motivation, and mental wellbeing. *Nurse Education in Practice, 51,* 102989. https://doi.org/10.1016/j.nepr.2021.102989

A study which recognises the pressures of being a student nurse both in practice and in personal life and focuses on self-compassion.

**Jarvis, P.** (2006). *Towards a comprehensive theory of human learning: Lifelong learning and the learning society* (Vol. 1). Routledge.

This book offers a broad examination of different types of learning and is helpful for understanding how and why we learn.

**Miarkowska, D.** (2024). *How to write brilliantly.* Sage.

This is a guide to the academic writing process, helping you to grow in confidence, to write critically and engagingly, and to develop your voice. Assists you into the mindset for independent study and reflection.

**Richards, H. & Malomo, M.** (2025). Empowering reflective practice. In *Developing your professional identity* (pp. 21–38). Routledge.

Specifically, for those working with children but contains useful information for all who reflect.

**Thompson, C. & Spenceley, L.** (2019). *Learning theories for everyday teaching.* Learning Matters.

This book provides a straightforward approach to learning theories.

**Vabo, G., Slettebø, Å. & Fossum, M.** (2021). Nursing students' professional identity development: An integrative review. *Nordic Journal of Nursing Research, 42*(2), 62–75. https://doi.org/10.1177/20571585211029857

A study which concludes that students need an environment with a caring and supportive atmosphere, so that they experience a climate for reflection on both practical and theoretical activities.

## Useful websites

**Honey, P. & Mumford, A.** (2012). *Learning styles* https://www.youtube.com/watch?v=2N3VjCzMYZY

A concise evaluation of this learning style theory.

**https://www.worcester.ac.uk/documents/4-Learning-Process-activities.pdf**

Activity 1 offers another view of learning styles and includes an online survey to help you determine your style.

**https://www.nmc.org.uk/standards-for-education-and-training/standards-for-student-supervision-and-assessment/**

The standards for student supervision and assessment set out the roles and responsibilities of practice supervisors and assessors, and how they must make sure students receive high-quality learning, support and supervision during their practice placements. They also set our expectations for the learning, support and supervision of students in the practice environment. As well as setting out how students are assessed for theory and practice learning.

# Chapter 6 Reflection and reflexivity

## NMC Future Nurse: Standards of Proficiency for Registered Nurses

This chapter will address the following platforms and proficiencies:

**Platform 1: Being an accountable professional**

1.17 Take responsibility for continuous self-reflection, seeking and responding to support and feedback to develop their professional knowledge and skills.

**Platform 5: Leading and managing nursing care and working in teams**

5.6 Exhibit leadership potential by demonstrating an ability to guide, support, and motivate individuals and interact confidently with other members of the care team.

5.10 Contribute to supervision and team reflection activities to promote improvements in practice and services.

## Chapter aims

After reading this chapter you will be able to:

- describe reflective conceptualisation at different stages of professional preparation;
- demonstrate how reflexivity may change your awareness in new ways;
- identify developing insight;
- relate to the experiences of others.

### Case Study 6.1: Gary: Peer support or collusion?

Gary was in the final year of his adult nursing programme. The cohort had been divided into study groups at the start of the programme and there had been few changes to Gary's study group of six students. The students were currently completing their dissertations and two of the group members suggested that they share their work to learn, get ideas and compare their levels of work. Gary felt uncomfortable and worried about the suggestion as he wanted to avoid any accidental or intentional plagiarism or collusion. Gary voiced his concerns to the study group. A couple of members were sympathetic to his views whereas others reacted defensively, saying that Gary was labelling them as dishonest. This led to an argument and Gary felt upset and disappointed as a result.

While out walking that evening, Gary reflected on what had happened. He was protective of his work because his final degree classification was important to him, and he did not want it jeopardised through academic mistakes. Analysing this, Gary became aware that he and his siblings had inherited a strong work and moral ethic by his parents and this had clearly influenced him. He wanted his parents to be proud of his final degree result because they had worked hard to give their children a good education. Thinking back on the situation, he considered how his reaction might have appeared to the study group members. He realised that he had, subconsciously, assumed that the study group members who had made the suggestion, and who had responded defensively might use the work for their own gain. Although this was an assumption, Gary felt that their reaction supported his ideas.

Gary called a study group meeting and apologised for the impression he might have given. He went on to explain that, according to the university rules, the suggestion to share their work could be considered collusion and he wanted to protect himself and the group from academic mistakes in the final stage of their programme. Discussing the situation and possible consequences calmly within the group resulted in consensus and agreement that it was, perhaps, inappropriate to compare work. As a compromise, Gary shared the reasons behind his choice of topic, how he had searched for evidence and what the recommendations for practice might be. The rest of the study group members did the same and they discussed any strengths and weaknesses they had noticed in each other's work. In retrospect, all the study group members agreed that this activity had been helpful, and each member had a deeper understanding of their topic and ideas for honing their work.

## Introduction

This chapter begins by defining what reflexivity is and then proceeds to offer opportunities for you to examine how you can influence your experiences and how those experiences might influence you. The focus is on the role of reflexivity in developing opportunities for learning.

## What is reflexivity?

In previous chapters we discussed reflection and reflective practice and, although reflection can be seen as a way of being – a way to learn from experience through asking questions – reflexivity is to turn back on yourself. Hertz (1997, pviii) suggests that it is like having *an ongoing conversation about experience while simultaneously living in the moment.* This is clearly illustrated in the story in Case Study 6.1, where Gary felt hesitant in sharing his work with the study group. This was not a conscious distrust of his peers or unwillingness to share his ideas; rather, his behaviour was influenced by his personal autobiography (as discussed in Chapter 3). This required Gary to examine the surrounding factors of how situations arise and in what ways his reflections might help him to influence his experiences, as well as how those experiences shape him as a person and a practitioner.

Reflexivity, therefore, involves a continuous review of personal action to enact change (Alheit, 2018). To do this requires you to examine your personal actions and assumptions within the context of wider social interactions. For example, you are a developing practitioner within a wider profession, which has rules, regulations and expectations of its practitioners but is also represented by those practitioners. In this way it becomes possible for you to open up opportunities to consider how you influence your learning, how you influence professional understanding and how this is influenced by life and social patterns. For example, how you study will, partly, be influenced by the ways you have found successful in the past, but also by how your peer group perceives the concept of studying. In Gary's example (Case study 6.1), his background had influenced him to be self-reliant in his studying. He experienced an ethical dilemma but came back on track because of fear of the penalties; however, this experience created assumptions about others. It is only through reflecting and being reflexive that Gary reached a different conclusion that benefited his learning.

Equally, part of reflexivity is recognising that knowledge and knowing are integrated with the self. In other words, knowing is not separate from you as a person and what you bring to your understanding at any given time. For example, the culture you grew up in influenced who you are and how you perceive things, as discussed in Chapter 3 and Case Study 6.1. This is part of a **socialisation** process that continues throughout life (Jarvis, 2007). Culture and socialisation may influence your perceptions of what is similar to your view, what is different and what is considered important. This will have been modified by other cultures such as school, university and working life and the professional culture and contexts of nursing will continue to alter your sense of self and how you integrate knowledge and knowing. Socialisation into the profession and its body of knowledge sets boundaries that become defendable when working with others (Geoghan Marold et al., 2025). Anxiety and overemphasis on results can lead to a tick-box approach when completing learning activities but limit actual learning. Consequently, reflexivity can be limited and superficial when other priorities take over. In Case Study 6.1, Gary is initially held back by such an attitude. Reflexivity involves 'mindfulness', which means paying attention to situations, staff conduct and practice contexts to monitor for potential problems and solutions (Noble et al., 2025; Iedema, 2011). Mindfulness will be discussed in more detail in Chapter 7.

## Activity 6.1 Reflection

In the light of Case Study 6.1, locate and identify the university's definitions of 'plagiarism' and 'collusion'. Make a note for yourself of differences between the two. If necessary, discuss the terms with a member of the academic staff. As registered staff, please undertake the same learning activity to provide you with the information to advise any learners you may need to supervise.

*As this information is particular to your university, there are no outline answers to this activity at the end of the chapter.*

Consider Case Study 6.2 to identify how reflexivity may become limited between teams.

## Case Study 6.2: Sue's experience of fragmenting teams

Sue was in the second year of the nurse apprentice programme and working on an orthopaedic ward. The ward next door was often short-staffed, and the qualified nurses from Sue's ward were frequently asked to cover. Staff on Sue's ward helped each other out by coming in earlier or going home later. They were resentful that the ward next door did not seem to do the same and that they often had to help them. Sue observed that this started to affect relationships and cause tensions. The hostile atmosphere also impacted on learning opportunities.

On her ward Sue observed that there were numerous learning opportunities because the staff constantly shared practice and reflected on what they were doing. The ward manager had set up a programme of lunchtime sessions where they could do this, and this included other professionals who came in to talk about their perspectives as well. However, it was interesting that the staff did not appear to reflect on the relationship with the other ward and Sue started to think about why this might be.

There appeared to be different cultures on the two wards. On Sue's ward, the manager was proactive to support learning and her staff. On the other ward, staff felt that they had little input and experienced less support. Sue came to this conclusion because one of her friends was working on the other ward. Sue wondered whether the perceived lack of support was why staff were reluctant to give up any more of their own time and whether this was contributing to the atmosphere between the wards.

*(Continued)*

(Continued)

Sue considered the difference in attitude between the wards in terms of being a nurse and what this meant to her. She had come into nursing because she saw helping people as a vocation rather than a job. To Sue, this meant that, if patients needed extra time, she would stay later than the end of her shift. Having been brought up to help people, Sue saw this as a normal part of her role. She felt she could understand the resentment of the staff on her ward, because she perceived the other ward's staff not contributing as much and sometimes taking advantage as they knew they would get help.

## Activity 6.2 Reflection

- Looking at this Case Study reflexively, what interpretations might you have?
- What area of commonality might offer the potential for the staff to forge a different relationship?

*There are outline answers to these questions at the end of the chapter.*

Case Study 6.2 may have helped you to identify that, even when we are reflecting, we often do not think reflexively about situations, how culture influences us and what this contributes to the circumstances we encounter.

By undertaking Activity 6.3 you will be able to develop some insight into how culture influences your reflexive thinking.

## Activity 6.3 Critical thinking

When thinking about the different cultures you have experienced at home, at school, through your friends and professionally, consider the following questions:

- Looking back how have various cultures influenced you?
- What is important to you in learning to be a nurse?
- How does your background influence your views of learning as a nurse?
- What kind of knowledge is important to you and why do you think it is important?
- How are you developing your self-knowledge? Do you journal, practice mindfulness or do you explore your personality traits for example, to assist the reflective process?
- How has developing as a nurse professional affected the kind of knowledge you see as important?

*There is an outline answer to this activity at the end of the chapter.*

Through completing the activity, you may have identified influences on how you perceive things and what is important. In this way, you develop awareness of how your thinking is shaped and how you can exert influence on modifying your thinking and circumstances. We now consider the process of taking ownership.

# Taking ownership

Taking ownership means taking responsibility for your own action or inaction. In other words, in terms of reflection and reflexivity, this means being responsible for examining issues and being honest with yourself in what you contribute to the situation, and what the outcomes say about your approach. By recognising your own participation, it becomes clearer where adjustments may be needed or may make the most contribution. The process of taking ownership involves:

- developing self-awareness;
- communicating developmental needs;
- using emotional intelligence;
- becoming historically and politically aware;
- informing yourself.

Personal insight and self-awareness are the cornerstones of reflexivity (Horton-Deutsch & Sherwood, 2024). Self-awareness relates to being attuned to what makes up our inner and outer worlds, how we think and feel about things, what values we have and potential contradictions between what we say and what we do (London et al., 2023). Superficial approaches to reflection and reflexivity are sometimes used as ways of avoiding ownership, because their instrumental purpose and limited analysis circumvent challenging the **self-concept** and, therefore, do not result in lasting change. The practitioner who has developed personal insight and self-awareness internalises these characteristics to become their way of being. Consequently, to continue learning, they remain alert as to how others react to their actions. Communication is, therefore, key; it is imperative to check whether our perceptions are accurate, and to explore the best way to move forward.

Although communicating developmental needs to others is part of the skills set, we need to build up during the nursing programme, it remains a life-long learning process. As nurses, we are expected to be self-aware about our knowledge and competence, and to address any deficits (NMC, 2018a). It is through reflection that such deficits come to light in meaningful ways, even if they were highlighted by others, such as a practice supervisor or colleague. You learn communication skills as part of your nursing programme, first by looking at basic theories in the first year and then learning how to apply these in different settings throughout the rest of the programme. Nursing communication needs to be therapeutic and professional in relation to how you communicate with patients, families, carers, and other professionals when organising care (Watson, 2024; Sharkiya, 2023). However, communicating our learning needs may feel challenging when we lack confidence, or have concerns about how we are perceived by others. Even experienced practitioners may fear acknowledging developmental needs and this can leave one feeling very vulnerable. Taking ownership of your needs is an important aspect of being a nursing practitioner and requires:

- seeking appropriate support and guidance;
- dealing with your emotions constructively;
- acknowledging and embracing feelings of vulnerability and discussing these with a practice supervisor or colleague;
- addressing knowledge gaps;
- undertaking independent study.

Nursing involves working alongside service users and carers or family members who are often distressed or traumatised by their situation. Constant exposure to distressing situations can feel quite burdensome and is known as emotional labour. Emotional intelligence, on the other hand, is having awareness of one's own emotions and being able to read the emotional cues of others (Junious & Cain, 2025). When starting the nursing programme, you may have been somewhat aware of your own emotional reactions but were possibly less proficient in reading those of others. As you develop through the programme you will find yourself understanding your own emotions better as you reflect on your reactions and behaviour in relation to your autobiography (as discussed in Chapter 3). Similarly, you will find that you are 'tuning in' to the emotional states of your clients and patients – in a way 'reading' people by recognising cues in their behaviour. In other words, these skills can be brought to 'reading' situations reflectively by 'tuning in' to the emotional vibrations that resonate through the situation, and the language that you and others use to describe it. Using emotional intelligence means being able to distinguish stressors and work that are emotionally meaningful and how internal values are aligned with these (Cheraghi et al., 2025). At first, your reflection will almost always be triggered by emotion, but, unless emotional intelligence is activated to read the situation and people's reactions, reflection will remain bound to feelings and not move forward to actual learning. Part of such adjustment requires being aware of what has gone before in order to be alert to cues in the present – as previously mentioned, this is a life-long learning activity that you will continue to perfect. There will be times that your 'reading' of the situation is inaccurate – remain mindful that this is not 'failure', but another opportunity to reflect and learn reflexively from the situation.

Historical insight is an important part of this process. For example, if you are aware that a particular unit has undergone considerable change in previous years, it will not surprise you to find that some staff may be resistant to further adaptations. Political changes have a profound effect on healthcare priorities and resources, and these are equally influential in how supported, or not, practitioners feel themselves to be. It is sometimes easy within reflection to make assumptions about situations and their solutions without a historical and political perspective and, where reflective solutions are unworkable, lead to further frustration. Part of guarding against this circumstance is to inform yourself of the background, context and surrounding issues of the situation to ensure that your knowledge is complete. Informing yourself may require some independent study and, consequently, time which will need to be factored into your learning plan. Consider the following Case Study to identify processes of taking ownership of reflection and reflexivity.

## Case Study 6.3: Geeta's experience of developing ownership in reflection

Geeta was in the final year of her adult nursing programme and working in an operating theatre. She was on her last extended placement and hoped to secure a permanent post as a theatre nurse after qualifying. Geeta had been in this placement for five weeks when a second-year apprentice nurse, Joe, was also placed there for a shorter time, as part of his acute care experience. Geeta did not really get on with Joe because she found him patronising, and it appeared that some of the other staff also did not like him very much. Geeta's practice supervisor asked her to help orient Joe to the theatre suite and the ways of working, because she felt that Joe might respond more positively to another learner.

Geeta found Joe very assertive, and he tried to take over things that she normally did. The patients seemed to like Joe because he had a good patient manner that put them at ease when they arrived feeling nervous. He tended to want to be involved in the most complicated cases, which sometimes limited Geeta's opportunities.

One morning, Geeta and Joe were working in the same theatre. Geeta had helped set up the instrument trolley with her practice supervisor, and she and Joe were now helping the staff with their final preparations. The operation commenced and Geeta and Joe were invited to view the surgeon's actions more closely. On turning round, Geeta noticed that Joe had accidently touched the instrument trolley and potentially desterilised it. Geeta had no option but to tell the scrub nurse, which she attempted to do as discreetly as possible. However, the trolley needed to be changed, and this caused a short delay that was noticeable to everyone.

After the operation ended, Geeta was working in the dirty area. When she was alone, Joe came in and told her that she had made him look 'really stupid' and 'how dare' she show him up? Geeta explained why it had been necessary to change the trolley. Joe replied that it was not up to her as she was 'just a student'. At this point, feeling attacked, Geeta said that she found his attitude difficult at times, a view shared by some of the staff. Joe later asked his practice supervisor if this was true and was told there were times when he appeared not to listen to people.

Geeta had to take a short break because she felt upset by this incident. On her way home she started to reflect on the experience. Geeta was confident that she had taken the right action but was less sure about telling Joe that other staff found him difficult. She wondered whether part of her reaction was due to her own difficulties with him.

### Activity 6.4 Reflection

Write down your answers to the following questions:

- If you were Geeta, how and where would you start to take ownership of this reflection?
- Which elements of the Case Study would you consider to be particularly important?
- Try to reflect on this as broadly as possible. You may want to consider issues related to interpersonal communication, organisational structure, responsibility, status, autobiographies of those involved, for example.

*There are outline answers to these questions at the end of the chapter.*

This Case Study may have helped you to think about your reflections using emotional intelligence to discern the perspectives of others better. Reflexivity means that we can judge the effects of our actions on others and the effects they have on us. We now consider the role of reflexivity in developing learning.

# Role of reflexivity in developing learning

The role of reflexivity in learning is how students or registered nurses orient themselves to learning opportunities (Bolton & Delderfield, 2018; Delves-Yates, 2025). Such orientation involves bringing personal knowledge to the caring situation at the same time as recognising what meaning is made from the situation and related knowledge. To do this requires:

- being aware of internal dialogue;
- embedding learning through integration;
- recognising the relatedness of knowledge;
- having awareness of nursing as a community of practice.

Awareness of an internal dialogue means listening to internal reasoning processes, meaning and decision-making. For example, you may be involved in an assessment discussion with your practice supervisor in which you are talking about how you communicate with patients. Your practice supervisor may highlight particular techniques that need to be used, and that you know how to use. You might identify that your interpretation of these techniques is different from your practice supervisor's and therefore you need to decide how to proceed. Throughout the conversation you will be aware of a running internal commentary and this commentary may either help or hinder the outcome of your deliberations, depending on how in harmony or divergent it is from your thinking and acting. This process is a part of developing and integrating your learning (Martlew, 2023).

In Chapter 1, we briefly mentioned Carper's (1978) patterns of knowing and that integrating learning means drawing together these different strands of knowing and knowledge gained through the complexity of nursing and life in general (Zander, 2007). The integration process involves reflection, including listening for the internal commentary, as explained above, in order to embed new information and connect it to the knowledge already in place. The connections are made through reflecting on what is brought to situations, what is taken away from them and how well things went. This is part of the process of integrating learning explained in Chapter 3. In other words, connecting the insights from your reflection with your internal dialogue to assess possible consequences of your actions results in knowledge being related, rather than simple accumulated.

Relating knowledge also makes it easier to apply it to different situations. For example, relating knowledge of different communication techniques makes it possible to understand how some might be more applicable in one setting than another. Similarly, relating knowledge of physiological effects of virus invasion on the body to knowledge of economic and social pressures makes it easier to understand contrary behaviours and the prolongation of infection. In this regard, theories are suppositions that develop learning when questioned through reflexive thinking. Without such questioning, theories remain dormant in terms of learning and, consequently, are not easily recalled or applied. Part of being a reflexive practitioner is to help develop theories through different applications within the community of nursing and understanding the evolution of theories and concepts helps develop a reflexive frame that allows us to question these concepts.

Nursing is a community of practice that shares a common purpose of caring for people. People function within a *community of practice* (Andrew et al., 2008) in the way they organise themselves and their lives. Nursing, as a community, offers the possibility to integrate practice with academic knowledge through engagement that questions both theory and practice (Andrew et al., 2008). As a developing nurse you embed learning in that community of practice through the ideas you work through in your university programme, self-directed study and practice. The capacity to be reflexive within your community determines how successful this process is. Collaborating reflexively within a community of practice helps the student, and the practice supervisor, to learn personally and as professionals. Sharing ideas in a community of practice helps all parties develop and ensures that practice is dynamic rather than stagnant.

Consider Case Study 6.4 to identify processes of reflexive development of learning.

### Case Study 6.4: Charmaine's reflexive learning experience

Charmaine was on first placement of the second year of the mental health nursing degree programme and was working in a supported housing complex for adults with moderate learning disabilities. Although she felt she had developed good communication skills from her placement experience in the first year, and the voluntary work

*(Continued)*

(Continued)

she had done in the local support group for teenagers with learning disabilities and special needs before starting the programme, she was somewhat uncertain how these could be applied in a learning disability residential setting. This was discussed on the first day when Charmaine and her practice supervisor, Jerry, had their initial meeting. Jerry reassured Charmaine that for the first week he would be expecting her to observe and support the service users with activities of daily living while settling into the new environment. Charmaine was not concerned about the practical skills but remained apprehensive about communication with the service users because she wanted to ensure that she provided them with choices and was able to communicate in an appropriate way. Charmaine observed how Jerry always had a laugh with those in his care and the easy therapeutic relationship he established with them. She also observed how clear his explanations were for them and for her when she asked any questions.

At the end of the first week Charmaine and Jerry reflected on the week's learning for them both. Charmaine told Jerry what she had observed about his communication style. Jerry in turn highlighted how valuable he found Charmaine's presence in making him think about the rationale underpinning his actions and helping him to develop his teaching practice through sharing learning and knowledge. Charmaine was surprised by this because Jerry seemed so knowledgeable. His last statement that 'there was always something to learn' made Charmaine think.

## Activity 6.5 Reflection

- What reflexive learning is taking place here for Charmaine?
- What is she thinking about when reviewing her current knowledge?
- What reflexive learning is taking place here for Jerry?
- Think about Jerry's knowledge base and how it is being applied to assist Charmaine and develop himself as a nurse.

*There is an outline answer to this question at the end of the chapter.*

## Chapter summary

This chapter has begun to define reflexivity. With activities asking the novice and developing nurse to consider how they employ reflexivity, the chapter offers opportunities to make sense of internal dialogue and cultural considerations within the wider community of nursing. Through examples of taking ownership of reflective and reflexive processes and what they may reveal, the chapter makes it possible to develop insight, increase self-awareness and consequently increase the effectiveness of the practitioner. Underpinning this with emotional intelligence gives you the possibility to read situations more reflexively and integrate this knowledge differently to develop caring. The importance of reflexivity as part of reflective practice will continue in Chapter 7 where we also look at mindfulness in relation to reflection.

## Brief outline answers

In this section, answers to the chapter's activities will be outlined and explained.

### Activity 6.2 Reflection

Sue's background had laid the foundation for her to view nursing as a vocation, but life circumstances for some people might get in the way. Equally, nursing is a highly skilled profession that deserves to be remunerated. Both sets of staff appeared to feel coerced into working in a different way, provoking anxiety and making it more difficult for them to think reflexively. When thinking reflexively, Sue might see that, if the situation of helping out the other ward continued indefinitely, they might never get the resources they need in terms of extra staff because the staff shortages remain 'invisible' to middle and higher management. Perhaps this could offer a starting point for dialogue between the two wards, in how they might address this in the longer term together, and so develop a more positive relationship. Talking in this way might also help them to share practice and, through this, develop learning opportunities. You may also want to reflect on whose responsibility it should be to initiate this discussion between the wards: should it be the ward managers, or should this come from the staff nurses and other staff working on the ward? Try to question your answers as to why you think one thing or another. From a different perspective, you may want to consider what the consequences are if it is considered 'normal practice' to work longer than your paid hours. How could this influence staff morale and team loyalty? Do the staff on Sue's ward resent the attitude on the neighbouring ward or are they, perhaps, dissatisfied with the culture on their own ward? Do they feel unable to voice their ideas due to their feelings of loyalty to their team and team manager? You may want to explore how *The Code* (NMC, 2018b) relates to this situation; for example, the section *Practise efficiently* (items 8.2, 8.4, 8.5, 8.7, 9.1, 9.2, 9.3, and 9.4) and the section *Promote professionalism and trust* (items 20.2, 20.3, and 20.8). It would be good now to pause briefly here to imagine the potential consequences of the fallout from this situation in terms of bullying and horizontal violence.

### Activity 6.3 Critical thinking

When completing the activity, you may have highlighted some of the following points:

- Home and school are likely to have influenced your approach to studying and learning in more or less positive ways.
- Learning the skills of being a nurse is likely to be a priority for you.
- Your background may have given you a view of learning as a nurse that differs concerning practical and academic contributions.
- Practical knowledge may be of greater importance than academic knowledge, or scientific knowledge may be a greater priority than softer skills such as communication, because this is the evidence base for your actions.
- Your knowing is likely to develop by doing, as well as through sharing your practice and reflecting.
- Developing as a nurse professional is likely to have identified the importance of a variety of knowledge, spanning the psychological, sociological, biological, ethical, spiritual, personal and professional.

## Activity 6.4 Reflection

In Case Study 6.3, we should be mindful of the roles and responsibilities of Geeta, her practice supervisor, Joe and Joe's practice supervisor. Before escalating the situation, Geeta, could have requested a meeting with Joe, and the practice supervisor to clarify accountability and what her responsibilities were. This could have provided Geeta with the authority to correct Joe and discuss his behaviour. Early in Joe's placement, he may not have understood the principles of operating theatre conduct. Geeta's reflexive learning should include how she prepared Joe for the theatre and what she could do to prevent similar incidents. In terms of *The Code* (NMC, 2018b), you may want to read the section *Practise effectively* (items 8.1–8.6 and 9.1–9.4).

Geeta should reflect on her relationship with Joe and the other staff, considering their differing developmental needs and whether these were discussed with their practice supervisors. This could have been clarified in the initial meeting if, for example, Geeta was Joe's practice supervisor as part of her own learning objectives.

Geeta may also want to reflect on her feelings towards Joe, such as jealousy or envy, and whether her response was driven by feelings of power, and was her response to Joe's mistake an opportunity to 'take him down a peg or two'?

A substantial part of Geeta's reflection needs to consider her emotional intelligence and if she is aware of her own emotional reactions (as illustrated above). Is she sensitive to the emotional reactions of others? How was Joe feeling when he entered the theatre environment, and might his behaviour have been bravado to mask his insecurity? Did Geeta take the initiative to discuss the situation with Joe directly after the incident and perhaps explain the rationale behind her intervention in terms of patient safety? Or, by waiting, was she hoping that Joe might 'know his place' and that she could reassume the status of 'senior student' as she had protected the patient from infection risk? Geeta should review how her feelings influenced her behaviour and whether she felt threatened by Joe, leading to her escalating the situation. Geeta may need to read about exercising emotional intelligence to inform her practice.

Geeta should also reflect on how she handles unexpected situations. As a final-year student, one could expect Geeta to be more resilient and not to so upset by a confrontation that she needs a break. She had taken her responsibility and had acted in accordance with *The Code* (NMC, 2018b). You could conclude from her reaction to Joe's confrontation that there had been a personal element to her response, hence her feeling personally attacked and not being able to rise above Joe's emotions and defuse the situation, using communications skills she will have learnt throughout the nursing programme.

Finally, Geeta should consider the theatre suite culture, where staff dislike a student but do not discuss it with them, passing responsibility to another student without clarifying roles. This raises questions about the learning environment's safety and openness and whether Joe will have a fair chance of succeeding.

## Activity 6.5 Reflection

Charmaine's presence helped Jerry to focus on the quality of his explanation for the benefit of Charmaine and the patient. He was also re-examining his knowledge base in the light of Charmaine's questions. Charmaine was reviewing her present knowledge to identify what adjustments she needed to make for applying it in this new care context. She was influenced by Jerry's communication style, which she viewed as a positive role model for practice.

## Further reading

**Conway, A.** (2021) *Emotional intelligence: A working guide on how to develop emotional intelligence and interpersonal skills in social interactions.* Independently published.

Although this book can be categorised as a 'self-help' publication, it does provide some useful and practical information on developing emotional intelligence, self-awareness, and resilience.

**Goleman, D.** (2020) *Emotional intelligence* (25th ed.). Bloomsbury.

This seminal book will help you to understand the relationship between emotions and cognition, and the importance of working with emotional intelligence when working with people.

**Goleman, D.** (2021) *5 Easy ways to boost your emotional intelligence.* Independently published.

Another independently published book that offers suggestions in developing self-awareness and emotional intelligence.

**Jackson, J.D.** (2025) Using emotional awareness to facilitate reflection in nursing practice. *Nursing Standard.* https://doi.org/10.7748/ns.2025.e12415

This article offers opportunity to view reflection not as a task, but the ability to deepen one's insight.

## Useful websites

**https://www.nmc.org.uk/standards/standards-for-nurses/standards-of-proficiency-for-registered-nurses/implementation-nursing/practice-learning-experience-case-studies-for-nursing-programmes/**

Useful scenarios to work through provided by the Nursing and Midwifery Council mapped to proficiencies. Suitable for students and registered nurses.

**https://www.nmc.org.uk/standards/standards-for-nurses/**

**https://www.nmc.org.uk/standards/standards-for-nursing-associates/**

**https://www.nmc.org.uk/standards/standards-for-post-registration/**

# Chapter 7 The reflective practitioner

## NMC Future Nurse: Standards of Proficiency for Registered Nurses

This chapter will address the following platforms and proficiencies:

**Platform 1: Being an accountable professional**

1.17 Take responsibility for continuous self-reflection, seeking and responding to support and feedback to develop their professional knowledge and skills.

**Platform 2: Promoting health and preventing ill health**

2.9 Use appropriate communication skills and strength-based approaches to support and enable people to make informed choices about their care to manage health challenges, in order to have satisfying and fulfilling lives within the limitations caused by reduced capability, ill health, and disability.

**Platform 4: Providing and evaluating care**

4.2 Work in partnership with people to encourage shared decision-making in order to support individuals, their families and carers to manage their own care when appropriate.

4.3 Demonstrate the knowledge, communication, and relationship management skills required to provide people, families, and carers with accurate information that meets their needs before, during and after a range of interventions.

## Chapter aims

After reading this chapter you will be able to:

- define and identify morally active practice;
- recognise the fallibility of professional knowledge and developing practice;
- develop some strategies to manage knowledge deficits, near misses and mistakes in your practice;
- understand the need for reflecting on the complexity of decisions and consequences;
- understand the relationship between reflective practice and mindfulness.

## Case Study 7.1: Pam's experience of reflection and mindfulness

Pam was in the third year of her nursing degree, and she was reallocated to an intensive care unit (ICU). She was nervous before starting in the unit and afraid that she would 'be in the way' in an extremely busy and stressful environment. She was apprehensive because she remembered how the Covid-19 virus had impacted ICU in the pandemic but could rationalise her anxiety. Pam was aware of her limited experience with death and dying and, although she was open to learning the skills to care for dying patients and their families, she hoped that she would be able to manage her emotions when faced with the reality.

On her first day Pam was linked with Grace, her practice supervisor. They met at handover, Grace explained to Pam what she could expect from the day, and gave her reassurance; she could feel some of her nervousness subside. Grace's caring attitude instilled trust and Pam felt she could be open about her feelings of anticipation and anxiety. She told Grace that she felt less stressed and was looking forward to being in ICU.

One of their patients was Mr Lee, a 70-year-old man who had been active and reasonably healthy before his admission; his underlying comorbidities, type 2 diabetes, hypertension, and raised cholesterol, had been stable and well controlled. Mr Lee had been admitted a few hours earlier with a severe acute respiratory infection caused by pneumonia. Conscious and connected to a ventilator, Mr Lee was able to follow commands and move his limbs.

The nurses needed to check Mr Lee's observations and assess his breathing and the need for sedation to maximise ventilation and Pam would observe Grace rather than attempting any activities herself. Grace approached Mr Lee calmly,

*(Continued)*

(Continued)

reaching out to take his hand; she ensured that she made eye contact with him and introduced herself. She asked him to squeeze her hand once for 'no' and twice for 'yes'. Pam saw Mr Lee squeeze Grace's hand twice and attempt to smile. Grace introduced Pam, explaining that she would be observing. Grace then asked Mr Lee how he was feeling and if he needed anything and explained that she and Pam would help him with his essential hygiene, always asking closed questions that could be answered by 'yes' and 'no'. During this interaction, Pam saw Grace glance at the monitor occasionally, registering the patient's vital signs.

While addressing Mr Lee's hygiene needs, Pam was conscious of Grace speaking to Mr Lee, always making eye contact, and using a communication style where he was able to respond with hand squeezes. When he turned towards Pam, she tried to communicate in a similar way, but she sensed that he was becoming very tired.

# Introduction

This chapter will begin by defining what reflection on practice is and then proceeds to offer opportunities for you to examine how you can respond to your experiences using the evidence base. The focus is on the role of reflection in developing and responding to opportunities for improving practice.

Case study 7.1 demonstrates the changing nature of knowledge, and why it is important to reflect on practice to be able to respond effectively to change and add to the evidence base. Grace used her knowledge of communication, but acknowledged the individual's unique situation, to guide her support. Her openness to adapt to changes in practice is a fundamental feature of the reflective practitioner. If we accept that professionals do not always get things right, we have a point from which to examine the effectiveness of practice by reflecting on what might be done differently. Equally, as those in our care are unique human beings, they may not always respond in expected ways and such issues need to be added to the body of evidence. Being open to change and reflecting on it allows practitioners to learn and develop. It is important for students and novice practitioners to acknowledge limitations within their knowledge and to take ownership of potential mistakes through reflection. This allows them to learn how to be accountable and reflective practitioners.

As seen from reading about reflection and reflective practice, self-awareness and 'knowing ourselves' are key concepts. Although the concept of mindfulness has been spoken about for several years, in recent years it has now become more mainstream and therefore introduced to the nursing profession (Figure 7.1).

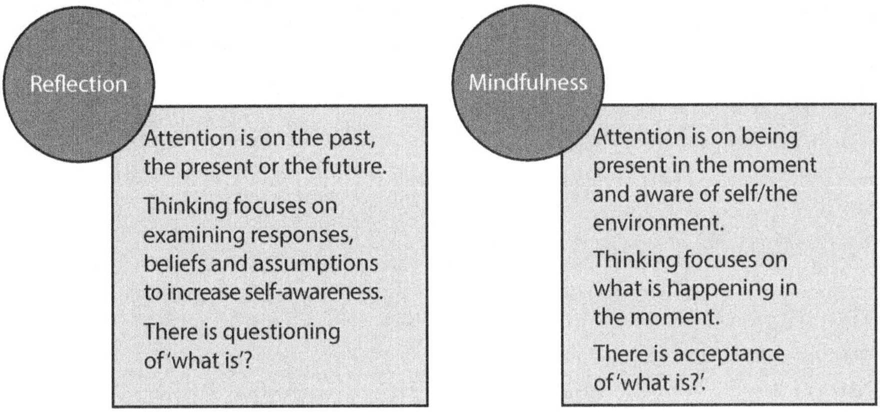


*Figure 7.1* Reflection vs Mindfulness (Delves-Yates, 2025)

Although mindfulness and reflective practice are sometimes spoken of as being similar, Delves-Yates (2025) suggests that reflective practice is questioning and awareness that contributes to (clinical) decision-making; as seen in the reflective cycles in Chapter 4 with reflection before, in and on action primarily used to improve and develop interventions and skills. Whist mindfulness is seen as self-care and acceptance. Johns (2025) applies an adapted approach to encourage us to reflect holistically on the patient/client and ourselves, in relation to the patient/client. This introduces new dimensions; in addition to the reflection before, in and on action, it allows person-centredness by 'seeing' all facets of the patient/client. In addition, we become aware of ourselves as holistic beings and, consequently, expose aspects of ourselves that may benefit from further exploration to develop as a nurse and an individual. This is the essence of mindfulness, as suggested by Taylor et al. (2015) and Nåden and Eriksson (2000, 2002) in which they discuss the concepts of 'confirmation' and 'encounter' as being key to the nurse–patient relationship. Clearly, there does not appear to be a distinct boundary between reflective practice and mindfulness; one could argue that it is a continuum between pragmatic reflection on an intervention or skill at one end, and a holistic (psychosocial–spiritual–emotional–physical) awareness at the other end.

Now consider Case Study 7.1 in terms of reflective practice and mindfulness.

## Activity 7.1 Reflection

There are two parts to this activity.

1. Now reflect on the case study and make notes where you think that Grace and Pam were being 'reflective' and where they were being 'mindful'. Include a rationale for your ideas.
2. Pause for a moment to reflect on situations you may have seen in practice where you witnessed reflective practice. Identify examples from all of the following situations:

*(Continued)*

(Continued)

- how interventions were carried out;
- how observations were interpreted;
- how communication strategies were used.

*Next try to answer the following questions:*

- What do you remember from the situation that caused you to consider this as reflective practice?
- Did you discuss it at the time with the person involved? If you did discuss it, what did you learn from the situation? If you did not discuss it, what prevented you from doing so?

*There are outline answers to these questions at the end of the chapter.*

This chapter links with another book in the series, *Evidence-Based Practice in Nursing* (Ellis, 2022) and encourages students to cultivate a reflective approach to their daily experience and integrate what they are learning through their practice. We begin by examining what morally active practice is.

# Morally active practice

Morally active practice is defined as critically exercising decisions based on ethical and moral principles and being able to justify these (Brechin, 2000; Buckley, 2025). The morally active practitioner recognises that there are situations where some influences, such as evidence and policy, may take precedence over others, such as personal values and patient preference, which might not be reasonable. However, some ethical principles (such as equity) must be applied, so practitioners need to be aware of the consequences of their actions (Howatson-Jones, 2023a).

Our moral thinking is influenced by the cultures we have experienced and our own histories and informed by professional expectation to accept and be compassionate towards others, regarding their situations.

We need to be clear about our motives and the expected consequences of our actions and be respectful of people's concerns and well-being. For example, we may have strong views about people smoking when they know it is harmful, and this may influence our attitude towards those presenting for treatment. Even if this is repressed, it may still be active within our thinking and reflections. A more extreme example could be when caring for someone who is an abuser, or a person who has inflicted harm on themselves or others. Equity means that care should be provided immaterial of personal feelings or prejudices. However, honest reflection on reactions to such situations is an important part of being able to deal with them, and of learning from the experience. Consider Scenario 7.1 and answer the questions at the end (Activity 7.2).

### Scenario 7.1: Morally active care

You are working on a busy medical ward. Many of the patients have complex health needs and you often leave the ward feeling exhausted. You are particularly troubled about the attitude towards a 26-year-old woman with a diagnosis diabetes. She has been admitted to the ward twice in the last 6 weeks due to binge drinking, which has affected her diabetes. Some staff within the team find it difficult to understand why she is putting her health at risk in this way. Nevertheless, you are trying to set aside background influences and see things from her perspective by chatting with her whenever caring for her. You do consider her hospital admissions to be avoidable and think counselling might provide a route to help her develop coping strategies.

You sometimes feel uncomfortable around your patient because of her lifestyle, but through talking with her, you have developed some insight into her behaviour. The ward manager has noted your empathetic communication style and asked you to write reflective log about this situation to share at the next meeting with all the ward staff to help develop empathy and understanding as a team.

### Activity 7.2 Critical thinking

- What is *The Code* (NMC, 2018b) likely to have emphasised about this situation?
- What might you have focused on in your reflection?
- What changes might you be thinking of making?

*There are outline answers to these questions at the end of the chapter.*

Morally active practitioners utilise a reflective rather than a judgemental approach to examine the outcomes of their actions and decisions. This means using your whole self when thinking about practice, engaging feelings and being aware of intentions.

### Activity 7.3 Reflection

Use the following questions to reflect on your own values and beliefs:

- What is important to you and why?
- What do you find difficult to cope with and why?
- Have the answers to the above questions changed during the course of your life and, if so, why?
- How have these issues related to your practice?

*There is an outline answer to this activity at the end of the chapter.*

Professional experience is helpful in providing the skills to develop, but also how we think about being a professional and interpret professionalism. For example, we negotiate the nursing environment freely, whereas those in our care cannot; this puts us in a position of power and needs to be considered in our approach to practice. An authoritarian approach that places us in control means that we may not see other perspectives that inform practice and are useful to reflect on. Equally, when we simply follow instructions and policies, we may appear to be professional, but without critically reflecting on practice, we are only conforming to established behaviours. This is not the same as reflecting which ensures the effectiveness and development of practice. Besides, policies and guidelines may seem to suggest that there is only one way of doing things, but nursing is dynamic and ever-changing, and there are few things in life that are more unpredictable than people. Case Study 7.2 illustrates this point.

## Case Study 7.2: Ahmed's professional experience

Ahmed is a final-year mental health trainee. Based in the community, he visits clients in their own homes to assess their mental health needs and ensure that all is on track in relation to their personalised care plan. One of his clients is 75-year-old Miss Sabire who has underlying diabetes with complications and hypertension but is on Ahmed's caseload due to long-term depression and anxiety. Miss Sabire has previously had acute admissions to a mental health inpatient facility due to suicidal ideation and attempts to take her own life. The mental health community team has agreed to call on her twice a week due to social isolation and possible loneliness that could result in an exacerbation of Miss Sabire's depression.

During their last visit, Miss Sabire showed potential signs of a chest infection. During the exchange with Ahmed, Miss Sabire stated that she did not want to be treated and did not want to see her General Practitioner (GP). Ahmed explored Miss Sabire's understanding of the potential situation with her and, with her consent, reported on the conversation in her notes. He also obtained her permission to share their discussion with Felicity, his practice supervisor. Ahmed explained all to Felicity and they agreed to visit the client together. During this visit Ahmed broached the subject of Miss Sabire's wishes, indicating that Felicity was present to ensure that he had correctly understood her wishes and had accurately documented the information. Ahmed also checked that Felicity was aware that no treatment could lead to pneumonia and a rapid decline for a person with a diagnosis of diabetes. As before, Miss Sabire repeated her wishes and Felicity agreed that Ahmed had understood and documented her wishes correctly.

A few weeks later, Ahmed arrived for his visit to find Miss Sabire in an armchair, breathless and sweating excessively. It was clear that she was very unwell and had an extremely high temperature. He immediately contacted Felicity to report back and seek advice, considering that the client had clearly indicated that she did not want to be treated. While waiting for Felicity to arrive, Ahmed tried to speak with Miss Sabire to ascertain her wishes in this new situation. Although she was very ill, Miss Sabire appeared to be alert and indicated that she understood the situation in which she found herself. On Felicity's arrival Miss Sabire repeated what she had just said to Ahmed; she felt so ill and breathless that she wanted to go to hospital and be treated.

### Activity 7.4 Reflection

- What do you think Ahmed has learnt about professionalism?
- What else might he have learnt about effective practice through reflection with Felicity?
- What options might they have considered?

*There are outline answers to these questions at the end of the chapter.*

When reading Case Study 7.3 you may have had further questions and thoughts about what was happening. It is for this reason that Nieuwerburgh and Love (2025) urge practitioners to reflect 'about' practice as well as 'on' or 'in' and before" practice. Practical awareness can develop only when such reflective thinking occurs and helps nursing as a profession to move forward. Taking responsibility for your own learning through reflecting about the practice in which you are involved is an important part of this process. We now examine how professionals may sometimes be fallible, and the role of reflection in managing this situation.

## Practitioner fallibility and reflection

As healthcare practitioners, we are subjected to scrutiny from several directions. The Nursing and Midwifery Council (NMC) (2018a) sets the standards for practice and regulates professional behaviour. The government legislates the policies with which healthcare is expected to comply (Department of Health, 2009, 2015), and the Quality Assurance Agency (QAA, 2024), through the *Code for Higher Education*, inspects the validity of teaching and assessment. With so many dictates for practice, it is understandable that professionals sometimes get things wrong. Human error theory asserts that mistakes are inevitable, but it is important to establish the reasons for flaws in judgement to address and learn from errors with the aim of improvement (NHS Resolution, 2025).

Activity 7.5 helps you identify some issues that play a part in errors and to reflect on how these might be avoided in the future.

### Activity 7.5 Reflection

Think of a situation where you feel you made a poor decision. Try to think of what might have influenced your ability to make judgements and decisions by considering the following questions:

- What were the circumstances?
- What was the result?
- What do you think contributed to it being a poor decision?
- What did you do afterwards?
- What do you think about it now?

Using your previous answers, now consider how to make good decisions.

*As this activity is based on your own experiences, there are limited answers at the end of the chapter.*

The decisions that professionals make require them to process information and use some level of intuition and cognitive aspects (Levy-Malmberg et al., 2024):

- Information processing refers to making sense of all the information available in terms of what is seen, heard, felt, smelt and read (Howatson-Jones, 2023b).
- Intuition refers to knowledge from experience being activated by the situation and inducing a response.
- Cognitive aspects relate to thinking about all of this and coming to a decision.

During the process of deciding, choices are analysed in terms of their possible consequences; we make a risk assessment, although sometimes we may not be wholly aware of this.

Social judgement theory suggests that the problem and informational cues link to the situation on which judgements are based. The ordering of cues, according to how we perceive their importance, determines how accurate the judgement is for the actual situation. The theory of acknowledgement relies upon remaining flexible and responsive, using information-processing skills to understand emerging data, allows clarification of goals, accesses guidance as appropriate and understands the extent and limits of our knowledge; these are all factors that contribute to safe and effective decision-making in nursing (Connor et al., 2025). This chapter links with another book in the series, *Clinical Judgement and Decision-making for Nursing Students* (Standing, 2023), and you are encouraged to look at this topic in more detail. Now read Case Study 7.3 and answer the questions at the end to identify factors that influence decision-making.

## Case Study 7.3: Elsie

Rose, a first-year mental health nurse apprentice, was working on a ward for older adults with cognitive impairment. One afternoon Elsie, who was quite confused, was missing from the ward and Rose helped her practice supervisor, Mary, search for her. Elsie was found sitting on the grass in the garden and Rose and Mary returned her to the ward using a wheelchair. As Elsie was cold, Rose helped her into bed, measured her temperature, pulse and blood pressure, and, under Mary's guidance, completed a clinical incident form. Elsie's temperature was a little low, but nothing else appeared abnormal. The doctor was informed of the situation and, as Elsie appeared not to have suffered any effects, told Mary to keep an eye on her. The rest of the day was uneventful and, although Elsie was restless and would call out every so often, she slept the night.

The next day Rose and Mary were on the early shift and found Elsie wailing; she had woken up in pain. When they removed her covers, they saw her left leg was externally rotated and shortened, a classic symptom of a fractured neck of femur. Elsie had not been out of bed overnight (she had a urinary catheter) so no one had noticed this deformity until Elsie awoke in pain. Rose asked Mary how they had missed this.

Bones of older adults are fragile because mineral density decreases with age, so even a minor fall can lead to a fracture. Sometimes the muscles encircling the hip go into rigid spasm and this, temporarily, holds the hip in reasonable alignment. When the body relaxes, as in sleep, the muscles no longer maintain their hold and the deformity becomes apparent. It is unlikely that Elsie would have been able to walk on this leg but, as she returned to the ward by wheelchair, this was not obvious.

## Activity 7.6 Reflection

- What contributed to practitioner fallibility in this scenario?
- What should or could have been done differently?
- What might be learnt from this situation?

*There are outline answers to these questions at the end of the chapter.*

Although registered practitioners are accountable for their actions and the actions of those whom they are supervising, students are responsible for ensuring that they report any changes or deficits they have observed. Reflection based on inaccurate perceptions can result in misguided decision-making. Schön (1987) suggests that when understanding is not grounded in proper practice through careful examination and checking of knowledge, inaccurate ideas about practice may continue because the reflection itself is flawed. Reflecting with others, as discussed in Chapter 8, and analytical approaches, such as those explored in Chapter 11, can help to resolve such errors. We now consider how to manage near misses and mistakes.

# Managing deficits and near misses or mistakes

Fragmented interprofessional relations can make managing errors difficult and lead to lack of quality communication between groups, creating working processes that are conducive to mistakes. Equally, anxiety can hinder progress because a person finds it difficult to make a decision for fear of getting it wrong and relies on being told what to do by others. Without the confidence and knowledge to question your practice, and that of others, poor practice and mistakes may be perpetuated, as the following case study illustrates.

## Case Study 7.4: Rhian's experience of poor practice

Rhian was a first-year, disability nursing associate trainee on placement in a nursing home. She had previously worked as a nursing assistant and was keen to make a good impression and do things correctly without appearing to "know it all". Several residents had continence issues but, during the day, through careful observation and trips to the toilet, they remained continent in a dignified way. Rhian noticed, on an early shift, that the residents had multiple incontinence pads in their beds that made their skin sweat and stick to them. When Rhian mentioned this to a healthcare assistant, she told Rhian not to interfere because this was the way things were done on the night shift. Rhian was unsure about this but did not want to make a fuss so decided to talk to Dave, her practice supervisor, and indicated that multiple pads were being used and that they were always very wet in the mornings. He said that it was different at night because the residents could not easily go to the toilet and so the pads were necessary but said he would investigate it. As the weeks passed, Rhian saw no change and felt uncertain and that, perhaps, she had been wrong in her assumptions. Rhian left the placement with the view that using multiple incontinence pads at night was normal practice. Three months later, when reflecting on another placement, she realised that what she had seen in the first placement was wrong. She decided that, if concerned about anything again, she would challenge the practice, talk to her practice supervisor, and follow it up with a link tutor.

The Case Study illustrates that, without reflection, developing practice and knowledge can be difficult. The Francis report (2013) highlighted the consequences of not following through on concerns about practice. Completing Activity 7.7 explores what you might do in a similar situation.

## Activity 7.7 Critical thinking

You are encouraged to look at your university and placement institution policies for raising concerns and then think about the following questions:

1. What factors would help you recognise a concern?
2. What might be barriers to raising a concern and how might you overcome them?
3. How could you consolidate your learning from thinking about these processes?

*As this activity is based on your experiences there is a limited answer at the end of the chapter.*

Like the case study, you may have recognised a concern about the uneasy feelings you had. However, this is not concrete evidence and reflecting on the situation and analysing surrounding factors (as we did in Chapter 4 with the different reflective models) can help you develop a strong evidence base. Developing reflective ability is a transitional process that involves struggle, accepting the challenge, making connections, learning to reflect more deeply and discussing with others, ultimately most of us strive to do the right thing (Nieuwerburgh & Love, 2025). Rhian could have progressed from her struggle with understanding and accepted the challenge of finding further relevant evidence. This might have helped her use the cues differently, make different connections and learn from the situation. We, perhaps, recognise Rhian's difficulty and challenge of questioning practice as a learner. However, with practice, this does become easier – communication is a skill and, combined with emotional intelligence, will stand you in good stead for the rest of your career. It is, therefore, important to start 'experimenting' with raising concerns and 'challenging' in a skilful and professional way as early as possible. It may be of some comfort to realise that *The Code* (NMC, 2018b) attempts to support staff who raise concerns because managers are bound by the section *Preserve safety: Act without delay if you believe that there is a risk to patient safety or public protection* (items 16.4–16.6). It is fortunate that Rhian was able to see 'normal' practice on her subsequent placement. Not challenging what you consider to be inferior practice because you fear recrimination can be difficult behaviour to change as a student, but also as a qualified staff member if you do not learn the necessary skills and communication strategies. Challenging inferior practice is an important element of *The Code* (NMC, 2018b); please read the section *Preserve safety* (items 16.1, 16.3, and 17.1–17.3).

Mistakes can be a 'shocking' form of learning through their abrupt nature. Similarly, witnessing inferior practice can also be 'shocking' because it is unexpected and contrary to ethical perspectives on nonmaleficence, justice, and equity, and is the antithesis of the nursing values: care and compassion. Mistakes and inferior practice can trigger an emotional response. Mistakes often leave us feeling emotionally upset and lower our self-esteem, and witnessing inferior practice often leaves us feeling helpless and experiencing an ethical dilemma unless the situation is resolved. Transforming the situation into learning through reflection helps us regain confidence. This involves considering how action, or inaction, contributed to the error, thinking about the nature of the mistake and what it means to be a professional. Responses can be categorised as emotional, cognitive and behavioural, as follows.

- Emotional response
  - Stage 1: shock and grief.
  - Stage 2: defence by projecting blame.
- Cognitive response
  - Stage 3: scrutinising own practice, acknowledging shortcomings.
  - Stage 4: scrutinising others' contributing practice to identify influences.
  - Stage 5: identifying the core problem and accepting responsibility.
  - Stage 6: checking core knowledge.
- Behavioural response
  - Stage 7: reflecting on the error and behaviour and how to change.
  - Stage 8: identifying how to improve and regain confidence.

It is important that we acknowledge emotional responses to difficult practice and errors from the start of our careers if we are to move forward to think about what needs to change. Now consider Case Study 7.5.

### Case Study 7.5: Roger's near miss

Roger was in the final year of his adult nursing programme on a day surgery unit. The pace of work was fast, with patients arriving and needing to be prepared for theatre. Often, premedication was required and had to be given quickly. One of the patients had been ready for a while and Roger and his practice supervisor, Sarah, went to get his premedication. They checked that it was prescribed and properly signed for by the doctor, that it had not already been given and that the patient had no allergies to the drug. They then checked the patient's name band and told him that the tablets they were giving him were his premedication. The patient's wife said that he had just been given the tablets. When Sarah checked with the other staff, she discovered that the patient had been given his premedication previously, but that the nurse had forgotten to sign for it because she was busy. Due to the alertness of the patient's wife this had been a near miss. Sarah and Roger completed a critical incident form for this episode and reported the incident to the unit manager.

When Sarah and Roger reflected on this incident, they felt shaken at the near miss and upset with the nurse who had not signed after giving the premedication. Roger discussed the merits of asking patients whether they had been given premedication already, but Sarah pointed out that they may not know what medication they had been given. Sarah highlighted that all professionals could make mistakes and that the only guard against this was to follow drug administration guidelines and learn from such incidents. They had learnt the importance of completing documentation correctly, in a timely manner, and of delegating tasks that might prevent such mistakes.

### Activity 7.8 Reflection

- What learning could Roger take from this incident?
- In what ways are emotional, cognitive, and behavioural responses evident in Sarah's and Roger's reflections?
- If you are an experienced practitioner, how might the unit manager have dealt with this incident and the nurses involved?

*There are outline answers to these questions at the end of the chapter.*

Regaining confidence after a mistake requires support as well as guidance to identify at what point decision-making becomes erroneous. We now consider reflecting on complex decisions to assist in identifying effectiveness.

# Reflecting on complex decisions

Practice experiences incorporate perceptions and interpretations that require action. The decisions we make, whether simple or complex, use a variety of subjective and objective data to reach a judgement. Subjective experience relates to how we experience our situation, is presented as a description and interpretation usually adds further subjective data (Price, 2024). An objective view, however, uses data that can be measured and recorded, such as vital signs and test results (Smith & Field, 2020). Within clinical practice, both views are relevant and valuable.

Reflection offers an opportunity to look for threads of meaning running through the information from a situation; analysing these threads of meaning helps to identify issues such as power/powerlessness and how they relate to the situation. The meaning of the analysis is not always immediately obvious, and reflection assists to extract the information required to read situations more accurately, develop personal decision-making and improve or maintain the efficiency and effectiveness of practice. Case Study 7.6 and the question at the end will help you understand these processes.

### Case Study 7.6: Natasha's experience of under-age consent

Natasha was near the end of her second-year nursing apprenticeship and working in the emergency department. A 15-year-old girl, Milly, was brought in with a suspected **ectopic pregnancy**. Natasha recorded her vital signs as per Paediatric Early Warning Score (PEWS) protocol and noted that Milly's pulse was raised and her blood pressure lower than normal. Natasha engaged in conversation with her while she undertook the observations and asked why Milly was so adamant that she did not want her mother to know. Milly confided that she always felt judged by her mother, who did not like her

*(Continued)*

(Continued)

friends and was very critical. Milly's situation would only confirm to her mother that she was 'no good', as she put it. Milly said that she mostly stayed with friends and spent as little time at home as possible. Milly asked Natasha to call her boyfriend instead.

After seeing the ultrasound scan, the obstetrician and gynaecological surgeon decided that she needed surgery. Milly was still clear that she did not want her mother informed. Her boyfriend was not interested in staying, saying he would 'see her later'. Milly went to theatre without her mother knowing and with Natasha accompanying her. Natasha, only 4 years older, wondered about the sense of this.

### Activity 7.9 Reflection

- What are the main issues within this case study?
- Who holds the power and in what way?
- What alternatives were available to the practitioners concerned?

*There are outline answers to these questions at the end of the chapter.*

### Chapter summary

This chapter illustrates ways to develop as a reflective practitioner. The examples and scenarios highlight the importance of learning from mistakes and offer opportunities for learning to challenge poor practice in ourselves and others. Reflecting to inform our practice enables us to recognise connections between events, how we are progressing and how issues such as power are important to the outcomes of decisions. The importance of sharing our reflections to develop practice within the wider profession of nursing is continued in Chapter 8, which looks at forms of reflecting with others.

## Brief outline answers

In this section, answers to the chapter's activities will be outlined and explained.

### Activity 7.1 Reflection

1. You may need to read the introduction again, paying particular attention to Delves-Yates (2025) explanation of the two concepts 'reflection' and 'mindfulness'. Remember, the concepts are not mutually exclusive and there is not a definitive boundary between them. For example, you may consider that Grace's actions were led by mindfulness towards Mr Lee; she viewed him holistically and understood that he might be anxious due to his inability to breathe independently, frustrated at not being able to communicate due to the endotracheal

tube in situ or he could be uncertain as to what the day would hold, due to him being easily tired. From a holistic perspective Grace could have considered Maslow's pyramid and realised that Mr Lee had a breadth of needs triggered by his admission to ICU. Grace understood a patient's need for human interaction to cope with the trauma of an ICU admission and to diminish psychological fallout from the experience; from her initial approach to Mr Lee, Grace addressed these needs. Grace's reflection on previous experiences of communicating with patients in similar situations meant that she first provided him with a way of communicating, offering him a degree of autonomy and the opportunity to be an active partner. She realised that explaining the morning's procedure would reduce Mr Lee's uncertainty, anxiety and feeling of helplessness.

Pam recognised the effect of Grace's approach from her personal experience. Observing Grace's interaction with Mr Lee, Pam became aware of the importance of viewing someone holistically and understanding their perception of the situation – in other words, Pam was 'mindful' of Mr Lee's 'being' and her own role in relation to his well-being. She used reflection-on-action to attempt communicating as she had seen Grace do but, sensing Mr Lee's fatigue, she used reflexivity and reflection-in-action to adapt her approach, not expecting him to use his diminishing energy resources to communicate with her.

2. You may have observed someone interacting with a service user or family member who triggered your attention. For example, this could have been the way in which an intimate closeness was established amid a busy environment, or it could have been how an escalating situation was defused. Was it something in the person's body language, tone of voice, eye contact or choice of words that you noticed? It would be interesting to find out to what degree the person was consciously choosing to exercise these strategies or whether this was a way of being. Carper (1978) would describe this as an aesthetic pattern of knowing. You may find it interesting to read more on this topic as numerous authors make the link between reflective practice, comfort, caring and compassion (another of the 6 Cs).

It is also interesting to consider whether you discussed this with the person at the time and the rationale behind your decision. In hindsight, did you miss an opportunity to learn from a good example that someone was (unconsciously) providing?

## Activity 7.2 Critical thinking

*The Code* (NMC, 2018b) is clear that practitioners should avoid making assumptions (please see the sections *Promote professionalism and trust* (items 20.3, 20.5 and 20.7) and *Prioritise people* (items 1.1, 1.3, and 1.5)). Taking these aspects of *The NMC Code* into account, you might have reflected on how background influenced prejudices about the patient. Depending on your knowledge base, you could explore possible reasons for her drinking and ways of managing her diabetes, and how these fit with information gained from talking with her. Also, you might consider how you could develop his attitude and communication style to become even more compassionate. You could discuss these ideas with the ward manager and develop a learning/action plan around these aspects of professional development.

## Activity 7.3 Reflection

You may have identified that honesty from yourself and others is important to you so that both parties can be relied upon. You may also have found that doing as you would be done by is a central value for you, so that you can be trusted. You may have identified that you find unkindness difficult to witness because of the emotional distress it causes. You could have become aware of changes in your values and beliefs between your teenage years and your working life, or possibly parenthood. You have possibly noticed changes since entering nursing. Changes often result from life experience modifying and altering our value responses, although core values usually remain. These issues may relate to your practice, how you think about team working and your attitudes to patients, colleagues, family and friends.

It is essential to be mindful of changes and how they affect you, your behaviour and your reactions to events and situations. Remember that most people do not experience in their entire lives the things that you have seen in the first year of nursing. It is inevitable that we change through our experiences, and we should remember to include those who are important to us in this change, otherwise we risk losing people along the way and perhaps even ourselves, as discussed in Chapter 6 in relation to emotional labour.

## Activity 7.4 Reflection

Ahmed may have learnt that professionals need to work closely as a team and that policy and guidelines are important for informing practice. Nevertheless, the patient needs to be a key player in relation to shared decision-making, regardless of what they may have indicated in previous encounters. His reflection could have highlighted that clients reset their boundaries when they are confronted with a new reality. Ahmed became aware of being able to adapt to Miss Sabire's wishes and, by being grounded in the here and now, he was able to choose the appropriate words to reassure her. During their reflections they might consider the power relationships between clients and staff or between different staff groups. They might also consider whether Miss Sabire's decision could have been considered invalid as she may have lacked mental capacity in the acute situation of being so unwell.

They may have thought about the following issues:

- the importance of engaging with the client, taking their wishes seriously and acting on them. It is a human characteristic to set boundaries under the influence of the situation;
- the individual nurse's responsibility when faced with a situation in which they need to make far-reaching and, potentially, life-or-death decisions;
- the importance of accurate and correct documentation.

Ahmed will possibly have an altered view of professionalism that is open to constant change and is constantly evolving to develop practice. It is understandable and correct that, as a learner, Ahmed should discuss such a situation with his practice supervisor. However, a point of reflection might be why Ahmed felt he needed to liaise with Felicity before reaching a decision about what to do. What would he have done if he were registered? Would he have discussed the situation with someone? In which case, who? The final stage of a programme is the most opportune moment to practise leadership and accountability.

## Activity 7.5 Reflection

Although not conclusive, factors impacting on our decision-making range from tiredness, overwork, stress and lack of knowledge but, also, disregarding the patient's perspective could result in interventions that fail due to non-adherence. Although we try to rectify erroneous decisions and rebuild our self-esteem, without reflecting on the quality of the decision and the surrounding circumstances, not all the deficits may have been noticed so only a partial solution may be put in place. Now explore what the NMC says about the factors mentioned above; for example:

- tiredness and stress: item 2.10 of *The Code* (NMC, 2018b) states the expectation that nurses need to maintain an appropriate level of health;
- including the patient in decision-making features in items 2.1–2.6 of *The Code* (NMC, 2018b).

Reflection helps to rebuild confidence and self-esteem and not reflecting often leaves us recalling the decision with shame, leading to a loss of confidence. When considering how to make good decisions in response to your reflection, you might identify that including others in the decision-making processes could help to overcome stress and lack of knowledge. Equally, including the patient could avoid non-adherence.

## Activity 7.6 Reflection

Elsie's behaviour was initially attributed to confusion, and since her observations were normal, no further action was taken. However, this situation should have been reviewed critically by asking questions, such as:

- What might have caused Elsie to sit on the grass?
- Is the way she is calling different from usual?
- What triggers and calms her?

A thorough physical examination should have been conducted to identify any signs that might have alerted nurses to more signs, which would have called for the doctor to see Elsie. Other measurements, such as oxygen saturation and blood sugar could have been useful. Nurses may need to review and justify their decision-making process through a patient safety incident form and provide statements. Students involved would also need to provide written testaments.

The key learning points include the importance of assertive decision-making and leadership, continual assessment focusing on the patient, and not relying solely on monitoring devices. Recognising changes in a patient's condition requires experience, open-mindedness and a reflective attitude. This is particularly challenging in long-stay or residential units with stable service users. Small changes in behaviour should not be dismissed, as service users are strangers, and their idiosyncrasies are unknown. This situation potentially breaches The Code (NMC, 2018b). Relevant sections include Practise effectively (items 10.1–10.4) and Preserve safety (items 14.1–14.3, 19.1, and 19.2).

## Activity 7.7 Critical thinking

Some factors that might cause concern are:

- feeling uneasy;
- seeing actions and behaviours that are contrary to what you have been taught;
- seeing negative effects for patients;
- inaction by staff to address issues.

Barriers to raising concerns might be:

- not wanting to draw attention to yourself;
- not being sure of your knowledge and the underpinning evidence;
- not knowing the process to follow.

Consolidating your learning might involve reflecting on your experience and writing a critically reflective account (see Chapter 11 for more information).

## Activity 7.8 Reflection

Roger learnt that mistakes happen, even with the correct checking procedures, when earlier errors have been made in a chain of events. He learnt to ensure that his documentation is carried out in a correct and timely way, and the importance of delegating if necessary.

Sarah and Roger responded emotionally to the near miss, with annoyance aimed at the colleague who had not documented correctly. Thinking about the incident, they considered their options. They thought that Roger's suggestion of asking the patient is not entirely reliable and could also suggest that staff might be incompetent. Sarah and Roger's responses were to ensure correct and timely documentation when involved in drug administration.

The unit manager should undertake group reflection with the staff concerned and develop this as refresher training for all staff to prevent such incidents happening again. Taking an educative rather than a punitive approach, the unit manager is likely to enable the staff to regain self-esteem and develop good practice. Another option would be regular clinical supervision for staff to help them reflect on practice in a safe environment.

Please read the appropriate sections of *The Code* (NMC, 2018b); for example, *Preserve safety* (items 14.1–14.3, 18.2–18.4, 19.1 and 19.2).

## Activity 7.9 Reflection

The main issues are Milly's serious clinical condition, her request for confidentiality, Milly's age, her mental competence and the rights of her mother. A possible ectopic rupture can cause major haemorrhage and requires immediate surgery. Since the Gillick law in 1985 (National Society for the Prevention of Cruelty to Children (NSPCC), 2018), doctors are required to assess the competency of minors to make their own decisions. If Milly is deemed competent and fully understands the facts of the situation, she may be considered competent to make the decision and give consent. However, it is for the doctor to decide whether the complexity of the decision is in keeping with the limits of consent and Milly's competence. A further challenge is an ethical dilemma between respecting patient confidentiality and safeguarding an under-age person.

Other alternatives might be to discuss and advise Milly to tell her mother, or to allow a member of the team to do so, or to inform another member of the family to whom she felt able to talk, but Natasha should be mindful not to superimpose her subjective experience on to that of Milly. The objective data of the vital signs and the ultrasound identified the clinical urgency, and Milly's subjective experience informed her decision.

As indicated, this is a difficult situation, so please consult *The Code* (NMC, 2018b), *Prioritise people* (items 1.1, 1.3, 1.5, 5.1, 5.2, 5.4, and 5.5) and *Practise effectively* (items 6.1 and 10.1–10.5).

For further reading on ethical decision making, please see another book in the series: *Understanding Ethics for Nursing Students* (Ellis, 2025a).

## Further reading

**Delves-Yates, C.** (2025). *Beginner's guide to reflective practice in nursing* (2nd ed.). Sage.

This book offers an introduction to reflecting on academic and clinical work and discusses reflective models in more detail.

**Ellis, P., Standing, M. & Roberts, S.** (2023). *Patient assessment and care planning in nursing* (4th ed.). Sage.

This book looks at different issues relating to the assessment and care of patients. It will help you understand and deal with some of the dilemmas that can arise in practice, and the role of reflection in helping to make your decisions.

**Johns, C.** (Ed.) (2025). *Becoming a reflective practitioner* (6th ed.). John Wiley.

This book will help you to gain an understanding of developing as a reflective practitioner in different contexts and through creative means.

## Useful websites

International Practice Development Journal: **https://www.fons.org/library/journal/**

This is a free-access international journal that publishes articles relating to practice development, many of which involve reflection and how to be a reflective practitioner. Type reflection in the search box to find a list of relevant volumes. You may even want to submit a reflection for potential publication yourself.

Nursing and Midwifery Council Fitness for Practise hearing outcomes: **www.nmc-uk.org/hearings**

Click on the hearing you want to look at and then on the outcomes for the details of the case. Reading cases from the NMC website will help you to comprehend the significance of justifying your practice and the importance of continuing to reflect on it to ensure your effectiveness.

**www.rcn.org.uk/magazines/bulletin/2019/june/mindfulness-meditation-tools-june-2019**

In 2019, the Royal College of Nursing (RCN) published a bulletin introducing mindfulness and 'the six steps to mindfulness'. You may find it interesting to access the RCN bulletin via the website and watch the films that illustrate the six steps.

# Chapter 8 Guided reflection and reflecting with others

## NMC Future Nurse: Standards of Proficiency for Registered Nurses

This chapter will address the following platforms and proficiencies:

**Platform 1: Being an accountable professional**

1.10 Demonstrate resilience and emotional intelligence and be capable of explaining the rationale that influences their judgements and decisions in routine, complex and challenging situations.

1.17 Take responsibility for continuous self-reflection, seeking and responding to support and feedback to develop their professional knowledge and skills.

**Platform 5: Leading and managing nursing care and working in teams**

5.6 Exhibit leadership potential by demonstrating an ability to guide, support and motivate individualism and interact confidently with other members of the care team.

5.10 Contribute to supervision and team reflection activities to promote improvements in practice and services.

## Chapter aims

After reading this chapter you will be able to:

- identify ways of managing the emotional labour of caring work;
- reflect in a group as part of action learning;
- reflect with other professionals;
- define guided reflection;
- understand clinical supervision frameworks and models.

## Case Study 8.1: Sally's experience with death and dying

As a second-year student on the adult nursing programme, Sally was on a hospice placement. She had been nervous about the placement and was unsure how she would cope with being in this setting as she imagined that the patients would be dying and it would be an emotional place to work. On her first day, she was surprised at the variety of patients and the cheerful atmosphere. The nurses worked efficiently, making sure they spent time with the patients. Jean, her practice supervisor, allocated Sally to care for Amanda, who had breast cancer diagnosis with lung and bone **metastases**.

Sally and Amanda had several things in common, including dance; Amanda had been a ballet dancer, but the chemotherapy exhausted her too much to continue. During their time together they exchanged experiences and laughed at each other's stories. As Amanda weakened, Sally became increasingly involved in her personal care. On her last shift Sally observed that Amanda's breathing had changed and told Jean that she wanted to care for her patient until the end. Jean explained that breathing changes often occur before death and encouraged Sally to stay with Amanda so she would not be alone, because she had no family nearby. Jean felt that Sally was ready to provide Amanda with her final care and Amanda died peacefully with Sally at her side.

Jean helped her prepare Amanda after her death, giving Sally the opportunity to talk about this final stage of caring. Sally explained that she could appreciate that some nurses found delivering care at end-of-life satisfying; she felt privileged to support Amanda. As they prepared Amanda, Jean asked Sally to describe the changes she had witnessed as Amanda approached death and after her death. Jean did this for two reasons:

1. It would help Sally to recognise signs and stages of death.
2. It would help her to disengage from emotional attachment with Amanda so she could leave the shift composed.

Through the process of preparation Sally felt that they had been respectful of Amanda and left the shift feeling sad but satisfied with her care.

Back at university, Sally was busy with assignments and course work. A few weeks later, when sharing this experience during a class, Sally realised how profoundly her experience with Amanda had affected her. The lecturer guided the group to reflect on their experiences, encouraging them to explore and analyse their responses and decisions, and what sense they were making of what happened at the time and afterwards. Sally realised that her reaction to the situation linked to the emotional impact that it had on her. She felt close to Amanda and was sad to lose that connection but also felt helpless at what Amanda might have felt at the end. Sally had used touch to communicate her concern and talked quietly to Amanda.

*(Continued)*

(Continued)

Emily, one of the class members, asked whether Sally and Jean might have been trying to control the situation, because Amanda had no way of telling them whether she wanted this type of communication. The lecturer asked Sally to consider how this situation might differ if she and Amanda were from different cultural and social backgrounds.

Sally was struck by the difficulty of determining what patients want during end-of-life care, because beyond a certain point care was based on nurses' assumptions, intuition and experience, and not necessarily on patients' wishes. This could make the experience variable for the patient if the nurses' assumptions were wrong. Sally thought about conversations she had witnessed about patients having a difficult death because they would not 'let go' and wondered about the accuracy of such judgements. She also wondered how she would manage in different cultural situations – a challenging thought as she considered different possibilities of this care experience. The process of reflection had moved Sally from an emotional position to thinking about her own practice.

## Introduction

Case Study 8.1 illustrates how reflective questioning from others adds depth to reflection and develops a wider understanding. As with Sally, questions from others can be confronting but skilful facilitation helps contain the anxiety that might surround such a process. As you progress through your nursing programme and career in healthcare, there are many opportunities to learn from others' experiences. This includes learning activities incorporated in the nursing programme and when working as a team member in practice.

This chapter considers how guided reflection deepens your understanding and analysis of situations, experiences and decisions, and how reflecting with others can offer support. This includes the importance of skilful supervision to make sense of changing roles and the challenges that healthcare professionals face daily. This builds on previous chapters, drawing on professional cultures and styles of guided reflection to identify how varying forms of reflection are applicable across professions, and how increased interprofessional working and learning contribute to shared reflective opportunities. The chapter identifies opportunities that exist between practitioners and how these might facilitate shared reflective learning and personal development to develop further understanding of practice.

## Managing emotional residue

Nursing leaves emotional imprints and can result in emotional fatigue or burnout and unresolved emotions are known as emotional residue (Lachman, 2016). When reflecting, actions and relationships are scrutinised and your personal identity becomes increasingly prominent as you develop (Nieuwerburgh & Love, 2025). Examining an event means that cultural, social, historical and psychological aspects are considered for example, what led up to the event, what groups of people were involved, their perspectives and interpretations and how we might be feeling (Seedhouse & Peuthrer, 2020). Learning can provoke anxiety and feelings of vulnerability by admitting uncertainty and being open to shift your thinking, and even to reframe your beliefs and values. Now undertake Activity 8.1, using the example in Case Study 8.1, to apply these ideas, to help develop your understanding.

## Activity 8.1 Reflection

Read the example in Case Study 8.1 again.

- Make a note of what you think are the main cultural, historical, and psychological aspects of the situation for those involved.
    - Are these different for the various people and, if so, how they are different?
    - You may want to consider the people involved in the hospice and university settings.
- Imagine yourself in Sally's place.
    - Are your perceptions the same or have they changed?
    - If so, how have they changed and is there a relationship with the stage of preparation you are at?

*There is an outline answer to this activity at the end of the chapter.*

Undertaking Activity 8.1 may have challenged you to confront your views and fears about nursing a dying person, and how different cultures think about dying. You may have questioned whether you were 'up to it' and you could have thought about similar situations that might be challenging. Shame and embarrassment are often experienced in the workplace and can occur within supervisory relationships (Nihei et al., 2022). For example, if you get something wrong or do not know the answer to a question, you may worry that your practice supervisor thinks less of you as a person and as a nurse. Anxiety can affect your confidence and make you prone to mistakes; in this respect, relationships that are supportive and secure enough to allow exploration of thoughts and feelings can contain anxiety to some extent. Developing a good relationship with your practice supervisor or colleagues is a joint venture and responsibility (Ellis, 2025b). Now consider Case Study 8.2 and answer the questions in Activity 8.2 to think about this.

### Case Study 8.2: Veronica's first day on a new placement

Veronica was a first-year mental health nursing apprentice, and it was her first day of placement with the community mental health nurses. She was excited about this placement because she thought that she might want to work in the community once qualified. Greg, her practice supervisor, welcomed Veronica and introduced her to other team members, explaining who they were and how things worked. He also explained what they would be doing that day.

Their first visit was to Harry, a 65-year-old man who lived alone. Veronica was taken aback by his home. There were newspapers and, what appeared to be bags of rubbish piled up everywhere, and the smell was overpowering. Greg checked that Harry was taking his medication, chatted with him and then they left. The morning was busy, but at lunchtime Greg sat with Veronica and asked her if she was all right as he had noticed her reaction when they visited Harry. Veronica shared her feelings of shock that anybody would want to live like that and asked Greg how Harry could get into such a state. Rather than give her a direct answer, Greg asked Veronica to think about how she maintained control in her own life. They then reflected on some of the possible causes for Harry's behaviour and how to support him. Veronica went home with an altered perspective of community mental health nursing but also felt supported by Greg; he had not been judgemental about her reactions.

### Activity 8.2 Reflection

- What are the main issues in this scenario?
- In what other ways could Greg further support Veronica?
- What else could Veronica do to enhance her understanding?

*There are outline answers to these questions at the end of the chapter.*

Case Study 8.2 helps you to critically review situations that you might experience as difficult. However, taking ownership of the situation and looking for solutions can be challenging and critically examining events may feel uncomfortable by highlighting weaknesses that you were not aware of. Non-judgemental supervision supports a trusting relationship and helps us with this newfound self-awareness, eases the tension of recognising our confronted identity and facilitates us to learn and change (Jones, 2023). Facilitating such learning is a key part of your practice supervisor's role but being open to developing insight is a key part of yours. We now consider how reflecting in a group helps to develop critical awareness and how this can be sustained through action learning.

## Reflecting in a group as part of action learning

Developmental journeys are made up of stories, some of which may be patient stories and some of which relate to the nurse (Bishop, 2017). Action learning is a process that reflects on real-life situations in a group of practitioners to develop problem solving and knowledge (Hopkins et al., 2021). It draws together knowledge, experiential learning and creativity to reach new solutions. An important element is the spiral of continuity, which takes learning forward and transforms it into action. Group involvement, therefore, is vital to achieve reflective depth, to consider a breadth of potential solutions and for encouragement and support. The roles of various group members are as follows:

- The session starts with the *presenter* proposing an issue and presenting it in such a way that group members can understand it, so the message needs to be communicated succinctly (in 5–10 minutes). To retain ownership, the presenter needs to be open to feedback and able to explain the action plan being taken forward at the end of the session.
- *Group members* ask questions to clarify the problem and offer reflective insights to possible surrounding factors and other ways of viewing the situation. When the group members have clarified any points that were unclear, the presenter moves to sit outside the perimeter of the group to listen and take notes. The group members then discuss the merits of potential solutions to the issue and reflect on possible consequences that might arise from these, to enable an informed choice to be made. They remain focused on the issue at hand (15–20 minutes).
- Normally there would be an optional *break* (5 minutes) at this point to allow the presenter to collect their thoughts.
- The *presenter* returns to the group after the break once they have completed their deliberations. The presenter then reflects on what the group has discussed, shares what they have learnt from listening to the group discussion and puts forward their thoughts and ideas for an action plan (5–10 minutes).
- The *facilitator* attends and observes the group process, adding challenge, reflective insights and support as required. If necessary, the facilitator summarises the learning and actions at key stages of the group process, to keep things on track.

Confidentiality is a founding principle of such group working; without trusting that what is discussed will be kept within the group, it will be difficult for group members to share openly. Consequently, when such groups are set up, they often start with a contracting exercise, in which the group agrees on the rules for engagement and individual and group responsibilities, with confidentiality being a fundamental rule. Being a group member means giving a commitment not only to keep discussions confidential, but also to demonstrate commitment to the group through attendance and contribution to the discussions. This helps to demonstrate respect for the value of working together. Non-attendance or non-participation means that the learning environment, necessary for individuals and the group to learn, is not sustained.

## Case Study 8.3: Matt's experience of action learning

Matt was part of an action learning group that had been set up in partnership between the university and practice. The group met monthly to share and discuss practice and identify their learning from this process. Matt was working on a ward for individuals with long-term mental health conditions, which he was finding under stimulating compared with his previous placement, which had been in a crisis intervention unit.

At this month's action learning meeting, Matt was invited to talk about his practice. He spoke about a person he had admitted with chronic depression who had complex health and social issues and was not cooperating with the advice they were given. Astrid, a member of the action learning group, asked Matt to re-examine the language he had used when presenting the case. Matt realised he had been talking about 'patients' rather than 'people'. At first, on hearing Astrid's comment, Matt became defensive and his response within the group seemed to mirror his attitude towards people in his care. The facilitator observed the group process and allowed them space to resolve the situation. This worked well, and the group was able to de-escalate the situation. The action learning group discussed what effect labelling might have on the people for whom they were caring and how they responded. In addition, Matt's response was discussed and the effect this might have on his experience of the placement area, and how this could be turned around. Matt came away from this action learning session feeling that he had actively learnt something about communication and that his emotional response could be due to his frustration with his current placement.

The purpose of group reflection is to consolidate and develop professional knowledge and practice. Active learning is something that happens when we examine everyday practice and consider new ways of working; this process may take us out of our comfort zone, but this is the essence of learning (McCormack et al., 2013). In Case study 8.3, Matt was asked to reconsider his everyday language about working and realised that the way he refers to people and categorises them is not person-centred. This is active learning because Matt recognises how he uses language and the possibility of changing it. He became aware that he should change his passive–aggressive, disinterested attitude on the ward to being proactive and discussing his learning needs and objectives. Connections that support the learner in practice draw on ideas of developing 'professional craft' which relates to us, as practitioners, and how we engage with developing our knowledge and skills base. While others help to facilitate our development of nursing knowledge through supporting practical and critical thinking processes, it is through actively learning with others that we consolidate knowledge, recognise our unique contribution, expand our skills base and develop confidence in our performance. Scenario 8.1 on the craft of nursing will help to develop your understanding of what this means.

## Scenario 8.1: Administration of an injection

You are working with an experienced staff nurse; who has been a qualified nurse for 20 years and has worked on the unit for 10 years. Today she asked you to observe her administering an injection as part of your learning to develop this skill. She starts by explaining to your patient what she has planned and to gain her consent. It is clear that your patient does not like needles. The staff nurse returns to the clinical room with the drug chart and checks it carefully, washes her hands and starts to gather the necessary equipment together. All the while she is explaining to you what she is doing, and why, and asking you questions. She checks the drug ampoule and carefully draws up the drug with no spillage and little air being introduced into the syringe. She expels any air bubbles carefully into the vial to avoid drug spray. When you both arrive at your patient's bedside, staff nurse asks you to talk quietly and hold your patient's hand while she prepares the area for injection. With swift, smooth, deft movements she swabs the skin, inserts the needle, injects the drug and removes the needle again reassuring your patient, who hardly notices the injection and this whole episode takes less than 10 minutes.

You contrast her fluidity with your novice technique when administering your first injection. Skin is tougher than appears in this exemplar, so the efficiency of her movements must be related to her expertise. The next time, you observe her much more closely to analyse what she is adding. You note her ease of communication, which relaxes the patient and immediately makes the insertion of the needle easier. This first step appears crucial to the whole process and makes the skill less task-oriented and more patient-focused. You observe the coordination between swabbing the skin, inserting and withdrawing the needle, and the attention that she gives to the detail of the patient's reaction and physical consequences. Patient comfort and procedural efficiency are both important.

Scenario 8.1 relates to the staff nurse's fluidity, developed from undertaking the procedure many times and from slight adjustments she has learnt each time in how a patient moves, responds and perhaps even flinches. The procedure has become second nature: she does not need to think about it and is able to explain and 'do' at the same time. This illustrates that the knowledge has become embedded (Gobbi, 2021). Importantly, her prime focus is not the 'task' but the person; the way she communicates is as natural as her injection skill. Identifying how your practice interfaces with others is an important part of developing craft knowledge; it helps to highlight what is special to the nursing role and how others can contribute to developing this knowledge in other ways. It is powerful to have a strong role model to whom we can aspire, but it is also easy for inexperienced practitioners to become uncertain when they compare their skills to those executed by experienced colleagues. It is important to be mindful that this is a normal process of development. Benner (1984) discusses this development in terms of five levels of experience and explains how we view an intervention as several discrete actions when we learn something new but, as we progress, we learn to see it contextually, as illustrated in Scenario 8.1.

So far, we have focused on learning from and with nursing colleagues. We now consider the value of reflection with other professionals.

## Reflecting with other professionals

Following the Francis report (2013), the quality agenda focuses on developing the whole workforce to provide high-quality care based on principles of quality, patient-centredness, flexibility, valuing people, clinical relevance and promoting life-long learning (Department of Health, 2008). Boundaries are becoming blurred, and teaching, learning and supervision opportunities arise for the novice, as well as the expert practitioner, as roles expand. Reflection is not just about what has been learnt, but also about how the professional is changing. This will become more apparent as the Fit for the Future: National Health Service (NHS) 10-year Health Plan for England (2025) develops new strategies, for example. As roles change and new ways of thinking become apparent, the implications for you as a growing professional are important as is how you develop reflective questions. Reflecting with other professionals can put this into perspective. Completing Activity 8.3 helps you to find ways of doing this.

### Activity 8.3 Reflection

Think back to recent practice experiences and consider where your practice interfaced with that of other professionals. Write a list of all the professions you have identified. Now consider what opportunities there may have been within these areas to share practice and develop learning.

If you are an experienced practitioner, consider also how you can develop opportunities for learning from other professionals for students and for yourself.

Now think about your university programme and list any other professionals with whom you learn. Consider what opportunities there might be to share practice and develop learning.

Review your findings and draw up an action plan for how you could develop or benefit from reflecting with other professionals. Identify what your objectives for doing so might be by drafting some reflective questions.

*There is an outline answer to this activity at the end of the chapter.*

The answers noted when undertaking this activity enable you to exert some control over your own learning and proactively plan how you can expand your knowledge of other professions and share practice. The interprofessional approach is important to open up possibilities and thereby enhance practice. However, for the novice this may be difficult and, where there are tensions between different professional groups, the process may be better supported by inclusion of a guide who can facilitate reflection. We now consider the role of guided reflection.

# Guided reflection

Guided reflection is defined as reflection that, through the questioning and insights of another more experienced practitioner, can get beneath the surface of experience. The guide helps the practitioner to reveal self-deceptions and their limits, as well as supplying support and encouragement to deepen learning (Johns, 2010). In this way it becomes possible to peel back layers of what may initially be perceived as routine practice to reach the essence of deeper learning underneath, much as peeling back layers of an onion intensifies the chemical effects of the aroma.

During guided reflection, practitioners are expected to confront self-deceptions and distortions of their perceptions. Consequently, an experienced and qualified person is required, and it is important that facilitation is supportive and well thought out, and that there is mutual trust between the guide and the practitioner. Facilitating containment involves setting clear boundaries and providing structure so that people do not lose themselves in unnecessary and irrelevant detail but remain focused on what they are supposed to be doing and experience a transformative learning environment (Froneman et al., 2023). The following Case Study illustrates how guided reflection is used to reflect on a critical incident. The aim is to provide the support required to deal with emotional residues and to develop reflective learning.

## Case Study 8.4: Jameel's experience of sudden life-changing injuries

Jameel was in the third year of his adult nursing programme working in the emergency department with his practice supervisor, Ricardo. They were on a busy Saturday afternoon late shift when they received a call to say that there had been a serious accident and four children were being brought in with burns. They had been playing with cellulose thinners and matches and there had been an explosion. One child had 80 per cent burns and the other three had less, although significant, injuries. Jameel helped to prepare the resuscitation area for the arrival of the children. He noted that they were not accompanied by parents or other adults; when the parents did arrive, there was a lot of noise and confusion and Jameel tried to reassure the parents as best he could. Jameel and Ricardo accompanied Bobby – one of the children who had significant face and chest burns – as he was transferred by ambulance to a burns unit. On their way back, Jameel asked what the future held for Bobby. Ricardo replied that Bobby would need many operations as he grew and would also need psychological support to cope with disfigurement. Jameel left the shift feeling disturbed about several issues related to this incident. He wondered why no adult had been aware of where the children were or what they were doing. He also wanted to find out more about the treatment options and potential outcomes.

The next day Ricardo met with Jameel during the morning break because he realised that Jameel had been disturbed by the incident. Ricardo explained they had 15

*(Continued)*

(Continued)

minutes, and he helped Jameel explore how he felt about the incident. Jameel found it difficult to understand why no adult knew where the children were or what they were doing because in his culture children were much more closely supervised. He said he wanted to find out more about burns and their treatment because this area was new to him. Jameel and Ricardo explored differences in culture and some of the social reasons why children might play unsupervised. Ricardo provided Jameel with references and links on burn injuries and their treatment and arranged to discuss these further with him at their next review meeting. Ricardo helped Jameel to see that, although he had not been able to get very involved in the initial care of the children, he had performed a valuable task by reassuring the parents despite his concerns.

This Case Study demonstrates the importance of guided reflection after critical and life-changing incidents such as these. However, guided reflection is equally important for reflecting on everyday practice to review what you do and how to improve it. Clinical supervision is a form of guided reflection that can enable you to do this. The next section explains what clinical supervision is and introduces some of the models and frameworks that are used.

# Clinical supervision frameworks

Clinical supervision is a practice-focused relationship with a professional that enables you to work through emotionally charged situations to release stress and explore and reflect on your work, to gain constructive feedback and affirmation of effective practice (Freshwater et al., 2007). The experienced professional is the supervisor, and the person reflecting is the supervisee. Clinical supervision is relevant because it connects with various forms of support and has a role within quality agendas for practice. It is a form of experiential learning that supports reflective examination of practice and planning of development (Zonneveld et al., 2024).

Variations in clinical supervision have relevance regarding the facilitation and tasks of supervision. These variations in using clinical supervision include:

- autobiographical reports from colleagues;
- vignettes from supervisee and supervisor;
- educational input;
- networking with other disciplines to share supervisors can enrich the learning process.

In all forms, support and clarifying boundaries of responsibility are crucial to achieve learning and to avoid doing harm through the clinical supervision process This is important because clinical supervision makes professionals think about their self-concept as practitioners (Robinson & Doody, 2022). When setting up clinical supervision, careful planning and identification of objectives and goals are important aspects to consider. Location of supervisor and supervisee should not be seen as a barrier as working creatively using technology such as **virtual meetings** or synchronous blogging, and ward meetings for experienced practitioners to provide clarification, are ways to broaden implementation. The managerial role in terms of actual supervision and caring for the well-being of the workforce is crucial to establishing an effective supervision programme that enables practitioners of all abilities and stages of progression to learn and feel good about themselves (van Ooijen, 2013). Whether considering your first qualified role or as a qualified member of staff, one of the provisions you may want to think about is whether the organisation to which you are applying supports clinical supervision to its staff. If you are already employed, you could consider how clinical supervision could be implemented or improved. Clinical supervision should not be an add-on but should be incorporated into existing forums such as progress meetings for the student.

Clinical Supervision Principles: Points to consider

- Clinical supervision supports practice.
- Clinical supervision is a practice-focused relationship.
- Clinical supervision should be developed according to local need and circumstances.
- Ground rules should be agreed to support openness and transparency.
- Every practitioner should have access.
- There should be preparation for supervisors.
- Evaluation of clinical supervision should always take place to determine influence on care.

However, clinical supervision is only as effective as practitioners' ability to be self-aware and have some insight into their own feelings and behaviours (Robinson & Doody, 2022). Key stages of the reflective process within clinical supervision include the following.

- *Self-awareness*: the process of getting to know feelings, attitudes and values.
- *Description*: the ability to recognise and recollect key events.
- *Critical analysis*: examining components, challenging assumptions and exploring alternatives.
- *Synthesis*: integration of new knowledge and identifying action.
- *Evaluation*: making judgements about the value of the experience.

Self-awareness is about the relationship you have with yourself. For example, are you critical of yourself, too demanding in your expectations or not demanding enough? Maybe there are times when your appraisal of yourself might not be accurate or realistic. For example, you may think that you know how to do something because you have completed the task in simulation, without realising that, because patients vary, your practice in the initial stages will need to be supervised by someone more experienced. This happens no matter how competent you feel. Expectations and self-appraisal are all implicated in the behaviour we exhibit, and how open to feedback we are. The skills and attributes needed for engaging with, and getting the most out of, clinical supervision include:

- communication skills;
- reflective ability;
- honesty;
- being open to feedback.

There are several models of clinical supervision, including:

- calling on an expert facilitator who has expertise in the problem area and can offer some solutions;
- one-to-one supervision where the individual meets with the supervisor alone;
- group supervision where a number of people meet with a supervisor;
- using a supervisor from another discipline.

Consideration of the model for supervision depends on whether:

- The issue for discussion requires an expert.
- Peer discussion could benefit all parties.
- A group holds similar concerns.
- An individual requires support.
- The issue is too sensitive to be discussed in a group setting.

Whichever is chosen, it is important to be clear about the aim of clinical supervision sessions.

Proctor (1986, cited in Hawkins & Shohet, 1989, p. 42) devised a framework that draws together the managerial, educative and support functions of clinical supervision. These are interpreted as follows:

1. Normative:
    - managerial function concerned with safe practice/developing standards;
    - ensures adherence to guidelines;
    - talking to more experienced practitioner who assists supervisee to work within these guidelines and meet standards.
2. Educational:
    - reflection and exploration;
    - enables supervisee to recognise strengths and weaknesses to develop;
    - relates theory to practice in a critical way.
3. Restorative:
    - supportive function of responding;
    - helps to understand how emotional involvement affects practice;
    - enables nurses to deal with their own reactions;
    - provides a workforce that can deal with critical incidents/problems.

Alternatively, van Ooijen's framework (2013) suggests that clinical supervision has the greatest benefit when approached as a developmental journey (Figure 8.1). The starting point is as a novice in the use and understanding of clinical supervision, but, as competence and knowledge increase, so practitioners become more independent in their thinking – which continues to grow with increasing expertise when engaging with clinical supervision.

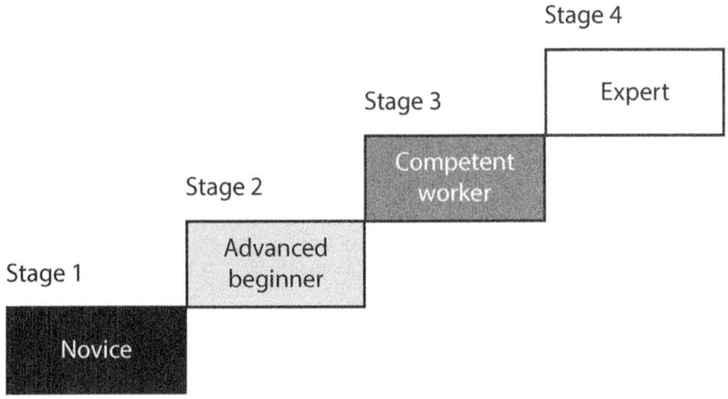


*Figure 8.1* Developmental framework(from Els van Ooijen (2013) *Clinical Supervision Made Easy*, 2nd edn, p. 18, and is reproduced with the kind permission of PCCS Books, Monmouth)

At the start of the journey, supervisees are highly motivated but lack insight and experience. As they progress to the next stage, they fluctuate between being dependent on the supervisor and becoming more autonomous. At the stage after this, the supervisees have more confidence in their judgements, and at the end they act autonomously, with the supervision process becoming a two-way process in terms of reflective learning.

Clinical supervision, as noted at the start, offers the opportunity to develop reflective learning and deal with the emotional residues of caring work. According to Faugier and Butterworth (1994), clinical supervision is:

- sharing practice-based issues in confidence;
- getting feedback and guidance;
- developing professional knowledge through reflection;
- letting off steam;
- acknowledging feelings;
- feeling valued through supervisory support.

What clinical supervision is *not*:

- complaining;
- unstructured sharing of events;
- personal/family matters;
- being told what to do;
- disciplinary issues;
- other colleagues' performance.

Undertaking Activity 8.4 will help you apply these ideas to identify suitable topics to address through clinical supervision.

## Activity 8.4 Critical thinking

List some topics that could be suitable to explore during a clinical supervision session (see the answers to activity 8.4 to help guide you). Start to reflect on the topics chosen.

How these might these reflections change during your working week.

Consider developing this work further by choosing a trusted peer to offer peer supervision.

*There is an outline answer to this activity at the end of the chapter.*

It is important to reflect on a suitable topic well before a clinical supervision session to prioritise what is significant for your learning. According to Driscoll (2007), a clinical supervision session involves:

- *preparation*: reflecting on the topic you plan to bring;
- *settling in*: the clinical supervisor will help you to relax;
- *down to business*: you will be asked to present your issue concisely;
- *clarification and summarising*: the supervisor will clarify what is important;
- *closure*: the supervisor closes the session with action planning.

As you will have noticed, clinical supervision is focused on your learning through the topics that you bring. It is also time that is dedicated to you and therefore something that is valuable and affirming. Making regular use of it as a healthcare practitioner can really help you to grow.

## Chapter summary

This chapter has looked at different reflective frameworks and ways of reflecting with others. The importance of others in stimulating the breadth of reflective knowledge has been emphasised because nursing interfaces with other professions and this can enrich reflective processes. Through the scenarios and case studies you have been given an illustration of possible applications, with the activities offering you guidance on identifying how you might proceed to incorporate some of these forms of reflection into your own practice and learning. How you start to record your reflections and write reflectively as another form of development is explored in the next chapter.

## Brief outline answers

In this section, answers to the chapter's activities will be outlined and explained.

### Activity 8.1 Reflection

Death, the accompanying rituals, and how people feel about it have different cultural meanings and are shaped by belief systems and personal values. These beliefs may be religious or historically embedded in a culture. For nurses, belief rituals and psychological aspects are key areas of focus. In Case Study 8.1, the cultural meaning for Jean lies in her belief that people should not die alone – a value historically common in nursing. Sally followed this belief, influenced by the emotional bond she had developed with Amanda. While Sally was more emotionally involved than Jean, Jean recognised the potential psychological impact and offered support, fostering an open and supportive learning environment.

Amanda's preferences are uncertain, though historical clues from her earlier conversations with Sally might suggest she would have wanted a friend or relative present. If Sally's culture had been significantly different from Amanda's, she might have struggled more and required additional support. This highlights the need to examine what we mean by "culture." Culture goes beyond ethnicity, race or religion – it includes individual values shaped by personal history. It's essential to understand a patient's wishes, but the connection described here goes beyond intellect. Turkel et al. (2018) argues that caring is a universal human experience that transcends cultural barriers.

In Case Study 8.1, it appears that Sally and Amanda shared values, and Jean supported Sally's decision to stay, believing they understood what Amanda would have wanted. Stuart (2022) discusses that nurses create a 'defence of self' to manage with grief while supporting dying patients. This protective mechanism also strengthens the nurse-patient bond and shapes how nurses experience death. For new nursing students, the psychological aspects may be most prominent, depending on personal history with death. With experience, nurses develop coping strategies and internalise professional norms. Very experienced nurses are shaped by their own nursing histories, which influence their reactions and the culture they foster. If Jean had early negative experiences with death, her response to Sally might have been less supportive. Instead, she was sensitive to both Amanda's and Sally's needs, helping ensure a positive experience of death and dying.

Pereira and Sousa (2023) in their research summarise what many nurses think: *it is an enormous privilege to be with people at the end of life.*

Elements of *The Code* (NMC, 2018b) are clearly relevant here – especially the section *Prioritise people* (items 1.1–1.5, 2.1–2.6, 3.1–3.4, 4.1, 4.2, 4.4, 5.1, 5.3, and 5.5).

### Activity 8.2 Reflection

There are three issues in Case Study 8.2:

1. The initial impression made by Greg's welcome to Veronica. This first impression has stayed with her, making her feel valued and supported, counteracting the anxiety of the visit to Harry.
2. Veronica's shock at Harry's behaviour, which clearly is different from Veronica's beliefs. Greg could explore these further with her but supports Veronica by sharing his thinking and decision-making with her. Veronica could enhance her understanding by sourcing information about the reasons for such behaviours.
3. They could discuss how person-centredness fits with a situation you find difficult to understand and how *The Code* (NMC, 2018b) can inform decisions. Please look up sections of *The Code* (NMC, 2018b) that apply to this scenario; for example, *Prioritise people* (items 1.1–1.3, 1.5, 2.1–2.5, 4.1, 4.3, 4.4, 5.1 and 5.4) and *Practise effectively* (items 7.1–7.4, 8.3, 8.4 and 10.1–10.6).

### Activity 8.3 Reflection

You may identify placements such as radiology offering collaboration with radiographers, rehabilitation areas providing access to physiotherapists, occupational therapists and social workers, theatres enabling connection with operating department practitioners, and women's health and day surgery arenas offering an interface with midwifery. Equally, during your orientation weeks you will have access to other professionals such as those working with children, mental health and learning disabilities. All these connections offer opportunities for reflecting with others through interprofessional meetings, reflective learning groups and case conferences. Equally, at university you may be involved in joint learning with other health and social care students, and this could involve elements of reflection on professional identity and the contribution from different professions. Your action plan might identify how to become involved in some of these activities the next time you are on placement. You could include listing which professionals have interfaced with your practice and what you learned from active participation in classroom discussions. Initial reflective questions might be the following:

- How does a different profession's priorities interface with those of nurses?
- What, as a nurse, can I learn about this profession?
- How does knowledge of other professionals influence my practice?

As an experienced practitioner you may have considered opportunities for students to spend time with professionals allied to your area, or you might arrange for these professionals to provide some teaching sessions in your area or student supervisions. The nursing role to initiate discussion with the interprofessional team should not be underestimated as nurses have always assumed the role of patient advocate (Gleeson et al., 2023).

### Activity 8.4 Critical thinking

The kind of topics that you may want to include could be:

- professional issues;
- exploring learning and development options;
- work-related interpersonal relationships;
- ethical/legal issues;
- work experiences, both positive and negative;
- skills development;
- managerial development.

You may have identified different ideas when reflecting with a peer and you may have been open to their suggestions because you trusted them. However, although such guided reflection is useful for opening up your critical thinking, you will need an experienced guide to reach any depth.

## Further reading

**Beddoe, L., & Davys, A.** (2021). *Best practice in professional supervision: A guide for the helping professions* (2nd ed.). Jessica Kingsley.

This book addresses the skills and practicalities of supervision and positions supervision as an activity for learning.

**Johns, C.** (2010). *Guided reflection: A narrative approach to advancing professional practice* (2nd ed.). Wiley-Blackwell.

This book explains guided reflection through a number of exemplars and the author's practice.

**Leigh, J., & Roberts, D.** (Eds). (2021). *Supervising and assessing student nurses and midwives in clinical practice: A practical guide.* Lantern.

This book offers a practical and contemporary resource to supporting student nurses and midwives in clinical practice.

**Woodward, S., & Bassett, S.** (2025). *Supervision, learning and assessment in clinical practice* (4th ed.). Elsevier.

This book explains clinical supervision primarily from the supervisor perspective.

## Useful website

**https://www.nursingtimes.net/leadership/what-is-clinical-supervision-and-how-can-it-be-delivered-in-practice-17-01-2022/**

This article explores different types of clinical supervision and aims to provide answers to some main questions about this process of professional support and offers resources for explaining different forms of reflection and for undertaking clinical supervision.

# Chapter 9 Reflective writing

## NMC Future Nurse: Standards of Proficiency for Registered Nurses

This chapter will address the following platforms and proficiencies:

**Platform 1: Being an accountable professional**

1.5 Understand the demands of professional practice and demonstrate how to recognise signs of vulnerability in themselves or their colleagues and the action required to minimise risks to health.

1.17 Take responsibility for continuous self-reflection, seeking and responding to support and feedback to develop their professional knowledge and skills.

**Platform 5: Leading and managing nursing care and working in teams**

5.10 Contribute to supervision and team reflection activities to promote improvements in practice and services.

## Chapter aims

After reading this chapter you will be able to:

- define writing reflectively;
- understand the principles of confidentiality and reflective writing;
- undertake personal reflective writing, such as keeping a reflective journal;
- undertake personal development planning;
- write reflectively in assignments as appropriate;
- record guided reflection.

## Case Study 9.1: Joe and Ross's confrontation

Joe is a mental health student nurse and is having difficulties with their practice supervisor, Ross. They have had personal issues that makes them feel unwell and needing time off sick. Joe phoned the ward and left a message for Ross. But, when they came back to work, Ross told them (in front of other staff) that it was unprofessional not to notify the ward that they were not coming in, and said it seemed to be becoming a habit. Ross said he would report this to the university.

Joe feels bullied and upset because, despite telling Ross that they had informed the ward, he still threatens to tell the university. This is affecting Joe's learning as they are highly anxious around Ross. Joe spoke to the link tutor, Elaine, who arranged a meeting with Ross. The meeting with Elaine and Ross clarified expectations of each other and helped Joe to explain that they had contacted the ward and left a message. Joe was able to say how anxious this episode had left them feeling and that they all need to plan a way forward.

After the meeting, Joe felt more positive because Elaine had noted that messages are not always passed on, so Joe felt Elaine believed them. Joe is not confident that Ross will commit to the actions of the communication pathway discussed. Joe is on edge around him and focuses on doing everything perfectly. Consequently, Joe is reluctant to try new things and expand their scope of practice. Joe describes the relationship with Ross as 'wary collaboration', which is not a positive learning relationship. Noting that Ross doesn't seem to recognise this, but Joe thinks that a practice supervisor should perceive the quality of a learning relationship.

Joe writes in their reflective journal, "If I were Ross, I would welcome my student back, ask how he was and then take them aside to find out what had happened. This would allow us to talk in a supportive atmosphere and help us manage any emotions. I have realised that, when qualified, I would like to be supportive, nurturing, and empowering. I want to discuss this with Ross at our next meeting, so have kept this reflection to return to".

**Practice supervisor reflection example (Ross)**

Joe documented the following for his revalidation, "I acknowledge that I often feel the need to get tasks done quickly and am impatient. I do feel guilty for not fully establishing the facts before confronting Joe. At our next meeting, I plan to check in with Joe about how he was getting on and explore ways to support him more effectively. I will also ask Joe and our other students for feedback on my supervisory style".

Recognising his own development needs, Ross concluded that he had much to learn about communication and leadership and would discuss his learning points further with his practice assessor.

# Introduction

This chapter explores reflective writing and includes ideas for registered nurses when writing their Nursing and Midwifery Council (NMC) revalidation documents. We may have an idea that reflective accounts are onerous and 'something extra' needing to be done. Nothing can be further from the truth if we see our reflective activities as part of a journey of discovery. There are few experiences more exciting than discovering how we think or feel about a situation, and why this is. Reflective accounts can offer us options and opportunities to experiment with creative ways of expressing ourselves (Fontaine et al., 2024) such as photography Dimonte et al., 2021), art (Leyden et al., 2018; McAndrew & Roberts, 2015) and poetry (Cronin & Hawthorne, 2019), with some of these authors suggesting that creative expression feeds the art of nursing, counter-balancing the science of nursing; the combination of art and science allows us to provide mindful, holistic and person-centred care.

### Activity 9.1 Reflection

Watch the YouTube clip 'Nursing the Nation', a poem by student nurse Molly Case from the 2013 Royal College of Nursing Congress. Take some time to reflect on the poem and note what the strengths and limitations are of using poetry as a medium to reflect.

*As this activity is based on your own experiences there are limited answers at the end of the chapter.*

The poem shows that writing reflectively requires depth of thinking regarding content and how to represent your ideas coherently and effectively. Besides allowing us to consider our experiences in a different way, writing reflectively equips us with ethical and analytical skills, allowing us to benefit from our practice experiences more fully. To do this, we need to look back on significant incidents, examine associated concepts and engage with analysing them.

This chapter explores the purpose of reflective writing in relation to the NMC Standards of Proficiency (NMC, 2018a). You are introduced to different techniques and encouraged to undertake exercises that help develop this skill. You are invited to begin personal development planning related to your reflective log, and reflective writing in assignments is developed in more detail.

# Writing reflectively

Writing about your experiences helps you to make sense of them, internalise the new insights, and contributes to your life-long learning. Reflection on experiences is articulated in different ways when we speak or write about them; speaking about situations is often exploratory as we put thoughts into words, whereas writing about circumstances is very powerful as we place our thoughts outside ourselves. Reading and re-reading our writing allow us to 'objectify' our thoughts and behaviour, and it is fascinating to experience how differently we view situations depending on our state of mind at the time. We often focus on unpleasant situations when reflecting, so reflective writing and re-reading these accounts help us view the situation retrospectively and from a less emotional position. We may feel uncomfortable about such accounts because of concerns with the presentation and what an 'invisible audience' could think of our ideas. It is, therefore, important when we start out writing reflectively that we manage concerns about who might read it, so that we are able to be honest and authentic in our reflective evaluation and writing about our experiences. Bolton and Delderfield (2018) suggest that, like Alice in Wonderland, we are open to uncertainty and new experience in playful ways; in other words, "to venture outside the firmly boundaried inner self into a place of exploration" (Bolton & Delderfield, 2018, p. 11). This links with one of the '6 Cs' – courage

- to include breadth and depth of thoughts;
- commitment to explore our thoughts and ideas;
- not be afraid of what we might find out.

Starting a writing journey means writing in formative and unfinished ways, first capturing our deepest thoughts and feelings as they start to surface. Consider the examples of reflective writing from the perspectives of student nurse (Joe) and practice supervisor (Ross), then answer the questions in Activity 9.2.

## Activity 9.2 Reflection

After reading the two examples of early reflective writing, answer the following questions:

- What is Joe's focus for reflection?
- What is Ross's focus for reflection?
- Are any further actions planned?
- If you were either Joe or Ross, how could you add depth to the reflection?

*There are outline answers to these questions at the end of the chapter.*

Reasons for reflective writing may vary, but the result is that you feel more empowered as you take control of your own development and learning, and you can come to a more positive view of difficult situations. However, the process can be emotionally demanding in what it reveals about you as a person and perhaps about others too. There are many reasons for undertaking reflective writing. These include:

- to log and record personal and professional experience and development;
- to help make sense of emotionally charged situations;
- to record other forms of reflection, such as guided reflection;

- to identify and plan career progression;
- to provide evidence of learning;
- to fulfil assignment requirements;
- to deepen understanding;
- for your own interest.

Read Case Study 9.2 to consider what opportunity it presents for reflective writing.

### Case Study 9.2: Faheed's experience of group cultural differences

Faheed was in the first year of his learning disability nursing programme. His peer group included a range of students from different backgrounds and professional pathways. They were studying a collaborative module that required them, in groups, to develop sections of writing reflecting on professional values and then present their writing to the class for peer feedback at the development stage.

Faheed noted issues with group dynamics when they were on a break and some students complained about the task and did not see the benefit of learning with other pathway students. Faheed responded, stressing the importance of professions understanding each other and collaborating for the good of the patient. He shared a personal experience of a family member recovering from serious injury with the help of different professions working together. The group began to see the relevance of the learning activity and returned to the task with more enthusiasm.

### Activity 9.3 Reflection

- What learning might Faheed take from this situation?
- How might Faheed compose his patch text about different professions working together?

*There is an outline answer to these questions at the end of the chapter.*

Group dynamics can be a strength or a weakness in terms of personal development and Levi and Askay (2025) identify that disruptive and aggressive behaviours arise from power struggles and a sense of competitiveness. This behaviour may result in a failure to control 'self' in practice, which has implications for those in our care and staff. Team relationships in any situation are always influenced by the personalities, psychological states and cultures of the people involved. Xu and Davidhizar (2005) suggest that there are cultural differences in communication patterns that can lead to misinterpretations and breakdowns; Western and European culture follows an individualistic pattern, whereas Eastern and African cultures favour group patterns. Group dynamics can leave students feeling disempowered and reluctant to share their ideas and needs for fear of discrimination.

When faced with group work in the classroom, it can feel demanding and challenging (Jakobsen & Sunde Mæhre, 2023). It is easy to become discouraged.

Chackal and Mitchell (2025) and Hover and Williams (2022) consider the phenomenon of workplace **bullying** and **horizontal violence**. Although it is not the intention to focus on less positive experiences of study and work, the case studies of Joe and Ross, and Faheed, do have aspects incivility and potential bullying. It is, then, wise to pause to consider the implications of this behaviour within a group as this could form part of your reflections and reflective writing as you progress through your career.

## Activity 9.4 Reflection

Now read the articles by Aydogdu and Disbudak (2025), Farrell (2001), and Hutchinson et al. (2006) and then consider the ideas you had concerning Activities 9.2 and 9.3. Perhaps you could jot down a few thoughts on the following points:

- How do you view Case Studies 9.2 and 9.3 after reading these articles?
- Have your view and interpretation of the case studies changed through reading the three papers? If so, please jot down how your perception has changed, and whether you would offer different insights and advice when asked to comment.
- Do any of the issues raised in the articles resonate with your experiences in either the university or the practice setting? If so, how did you address the issues when they arose, and could you address the situation differently after reading these articles?

*This activity is based on your reading the suggested articles. The full references can be found at the end of the chapter. As this is your own reflection, there is no outline answer.*

Wherever we work, we will always need to adapt to people from different cultures for us to communicate effectively. We should be mindful that, when talking about cultures, we do not always refer to ethnicity, language, religion, etc., but should also be aware that profession, gender, gender identity, age, sexual orientation, geographical location, for example are all elements of culture that could result in different ideas and behaviour. Part of our professional duty is to bridge these divides and develop learning opportunities. Curiosity and reflection about difference, commonality and inclusion are core concepts in interpersonal communication, respect and acceptance – accepting and respecting 'the other' means first accepting and respecting 'self'. We can develop in this area by continued reflection on what is happening, potential reasons why and considering alternatives. Writing reflectively helps us deal with these situations and with the implementation of ideas and is a powerful way of gaining **empowerment**. However, as our experiences inevitably involve others, it is important, within our reflective writing, to recognise personal responsibility and accountability to maintain anonymity and confidentiality. We consider this in more detail in the next section.

# The principles of confidentiality in reflective writing

Confidentiality is a key ethical issue in professional practice in terms of what is written and discussed (NMC, 2018a). Patient confidentiality is prioritised, but corporate confidentiality is not always considered. The Caldicott Committee recommended that all items of information relating to an individual should be treated as potentially capable of identifying them and be appropriately protected to safeguard confidentiality (Department of Health, 1997). Confidentiality means keeping information private. Corporate confidentiality means that institutions and organisations are also entitled to have their business kept private. This may be achieved by using a pseudonym and removal of any identifiers of the issues being written about. It is important when using someone else's information (such as a patient's case) to gain their consent for its use (NMC, 2018b).

Some authors raise concerns about the morality of using interpreted information about someone as a learning resource (McCarthy et al., 2016). This applies to information about clients or others, when writing reflectively, and creates a professional conduct issue and an ethical dilemma. One method is to 'bracket' identifiers and focus on the core issues; removing all descriptors that cause distraction allows foundation issues to emerge and be analysed. John's (2013) framework offers an alternative by examining background philosophy, theory and problem presentation, and the interpretation of reality, role and self-awareness through questioning, eliminating the need for descriptors. Background philosophy relates to which values and beliefs may be present in assumptions made about the problem, whereas theory is about the frameworks that surround our thinking about the problem. These are both used in how we present a problem and how we interpret our reality of the problem. Questioning our own role reflectively and developing self-awareness in relation to the problem is necessary, and this might be a useful model to try.

### Activity 9.5 Reflection

Revisit John's (2013) Model for Structured Reflection that we discussed in Chapter 4 and, using his questions of philosophy, theory, problem presentation, interpretation of reality, role and self-awareness, write a reflective account of the episode relating to your practice that you identified in Activity 9.4.

*As this activity relates to your practice, there is no outline answer at the end of the chapter.*

Please be mindful that when using student and client knowledge we need to be ethically considerate and sensitive, focusing on issues in an evaluative and analytical manner, and examining personal parameters of our responsibility. This applies not only to reflections on clinical experiences, but also classroom discussions, group work or any other joint activity. We need to consider this when writing reflectively, regardless of whether your writing will be seen by others. It is advisable not to focus on others in your reflections because they are not present to argue their case or discuss issues with you in person; it is better to focus on issues, rather than people, and how an issue affected *you* and how *you* addressed it. This means that others' confidentiality is assured and that your and their professional roles are ethically protected, you should strengthen this by writing a confidentiality statement to support your reflective piece (NMC, 2018a).

Read Case Study 9.3 and answer the questions in Activity 9.6, to help you think of how you might approach these issues.

### Case Study 9.3: Mia's reflection on collaborative learning

Mia, a registered nurse who had trained overseas, works in a renal unit where two third-year nurses, Josh and Ray, are placed. Mia had started an academic development course, which included how to search for information and complete academic assignments before registering for a practice supervisor/practice assessor programme. She had completed formative work reflecting on what she had learnt on the programme so far, but the feedback from her tutor indicated that her failure was because she had not maintained confidentiality or reflected adequately. Mia was confused and worried about **losing face** with her tutor; she was having difficulty grasping the principles of reflection (something she was not used to because she had completed an exam-based course for her basic nursing education). In the formative work she had described her learning and what she wanted to do, identifying the type of unit she worked in, the trust and where she was studying, but she had not named any of the patients.

Mia approached Josh to explain how he reflected so that she could understand where she was going wrong. He asked Mia to think back on how she felt when she started in the unit and how she felt about it now. As she described how she felt from different time perspectives, Josh asked her various questions, which he wrote down with her answers. At the end he asked Mia to read back what he had recorded from their dialogue. Mia was amazed at how Josh had captured her experience in a few words, but also how the questions had made her think differently about things. She decided to write about this process that evening and asked Josh for feedback on it the next day.

Mia rewrote the piece of dialogue by including how she felt her knowledge had changed and how building relationships with people had made things easier. She was careful not to include Josh's name, but to focus on the issue of developing knowledge through working and learning collaboratively with students. Mia included some critical points on how her arrival could have been facilitated better.

After reading her account, Josh made a few comments and identified a book that Mia might find helpful to inform her thinking about reflection. Mia felt more affirmed through this experience.

### Activity 9.6 Reflection

- In Case Study 9.3, how did Mia breach confidentiality within her formative piece of writing?
- What might be the consequences for her and what might be the consequences for Josh if he breached confidentiality in a similar way in his written work?

*There are outline answers to these questions at the end of the chapter.*

Collaborative learning between qualified staff and students is a valuable process. This is especially useful when considering issues of ethics and confidentiality; these help the student understand the parameters of accountability and why practice supervisors might see situations differently. Leaving out all descriptors could result in losing the situational context, so realistic description with patient or colleague consent might be a more reliable and ethical option. Remember to include that you have obtained patient or colleague consent in your reflective account; it is unusual and difficult to obtain corporate consent, which means that any identifiable markers relating to the healthcare provider or educational institution need to be removed. Also, even with patient or colleague consent, you need to anonymise anyone you include in your work.

We now consider personal reflective writing as a part of this process.

## Personal reflective writing

Reflection in nursing has a dual function: supporting learning and supporting the individual. It requires confidence and courage to acknowledge limitations and deficits, and a degree of insight to admit these to ourselves. According to Bolton and Delderfield (2018 and, p. 116) and Mahon and O'Neill (2020), 'through the mirror' (this relates to the Alice in Wonderland analogy in the Writing reflectively section earlier in this chapter) writing can facilitate deeper learning through:

- gaining perspective;
- giving confidential and relatively safe access;
- releasing power to take more responsibility for actions;
- using narrative to offer accurate observation, metaphor and critique.

From a 'through the mirror' perspective, writing is always evolving and may generate unexpected ideas. For example, when thinking about what caring means to you, you might remember when you were last ill and how wretched and unwell you felt. You might *feel* the rumpled sheets and the resulting discomfort, the clamminess of the temperature and how lonely you felt because everyone was involved in their own lives. This might stimulate you to revise your ideas around caring and think about what it means to you from a more personal perspective.

Returning to the theme of using art forms, as introduced in Activity 9.1, a medium such as poetry could increase fluidity of expression and help deal with difficult emotions by creating **cathartic** expression through the writing. Some people find it helpful to create a collage of pictures, cut out from magazines, which symbolise their ideas and/or feelings and then, once these have been visually portrayed, to write about the issue on which they need to focus. Other people use photography, painting, dance and movement to express their ideas and emotions and, in doing this, make their abstract thoughts more tangible before writing them down (McCarthy et al., 2016). Writing in this way can be exciting and empowering; you can develop different ways of formulating your ideas to make sense of your personal experience and, in doing so, gain control of the emotions and the issues focused on in the reflection.

Coleman and Willis (2015) invite the reflective writer to find new forms of expression. Empowering ourselves requires coming to know ourselves as being more than a professional identity (think of the personal biography that we explored in Chapter 3). It is in knowing ourselves that we can come to know our 'becoming' as well (Chan & Schwind, 2006). Poetic expression can express a unique part of who we are and does not necessarily need to follow rules. Rather, it provides opportunities for the playfulness described earlier in this chapter by Bolton and Delderfield (2018) as an essential part of *going through the mirror*, rather than becoming fixated with its surface. Poetry may not be something with which you feel comfortable, and it is not essential to use this form of expression; but experiment with it and you may surprise yourself. Remember, no one needs to see your writing. An example of poetry follows.

*What do you see when you look at me?*

*A caring nurse or a man alone;*

*What do you see when you look at me?*

*A capable helper or someone losing his home;*

*What do you see when you look at me?*

*Someone missing class or trying to phone;*

*What do you see when you look at me?*

*See the person, see the problem, see ME.*

*(Anonymous)*

This could have been how Joe might have started writing about his frustration in the student reflection earlier. The next activity offers you an opportunity to express yourself differently.

## Activity 9.7 Reflection

Think of something relating to your personal development that is very significant to you. Spend a little time reflecting on the situation or issue. Now try to write a

*(Continued)*

(Continued)

reflection about it using one (or more) of the creative suggestions suggested earlier in the chapter. Reread this and consider what response and insights this form of expression elicits.

*As this activity is based on your personal experiences, there is an outline answer to only part of this activity at the end of the chapter.*

Personal writing is often private, like a diary, capturing your deepest thoughts, feelings and reflections on your experiences. While similar, it differs slightly from a reflective journal, which will be explored next. Although reflective writing can be cathartic and **catalytic**, helping you let go of your emotions and achieve deep exploration (Driscoll, 2007), there also needs to be reflection on how your role develops as healthcare progresses and you develop professionally throughout your career. Logging reflective entries within a reflective journal helps keep track of what you are learning and your practice experiences, including those encountered during your preparation programme. In addition, consistent writing helps you to consider assessment, feedback and practice in terms of your whole experience and can, therefore, be a powerful way to integrate theory and practice. This approach, often introduced as part of the nursing programme, is imperative to professional life-long learning and is used in maintaining a professional portfolio and revalidation as a registered nurse (NMC, 2019).

## Example of a reflective log entry

I took on teaching a course that was new to me, and the first session had gone well. However, by the third session the students were confused by the advice I was giving them. I checked with the module leader regarding the assignment, but I found their explanation as vague as the written guidelines. Several students emailed the module leader directly and I was copied into the replies, which gave some clarity. At the next session I was able to provide concrete examples of what they might want to write about. Ultimately, my teaching of this aspect of the module was badly evaluated, which was disappointing.

**Main points identified from reflection on the experience**

- When I agreed to teach on the module, I was not proactive and did not ensure that I understood what the learning outcomes for the module were and how the assessment related to the outcomes.
- I did not communicate my understanding clearly to the module leader when I asked for advice on the guidelines. I should have asked for further clarification.
- I did not tell the students at the start that this was the first time I was teaching the module. I should have done this because, in hindsight, we could have worked better together to clarify the guidelines with the module leader. Using the knowledge of other, experienced tutors of the module would also have been helpful.

**Learning points**

- I need to be prepared to ask for help from both colleagues and students, to work together.
- I need to be open to identifying alternative strategies, which could aid learning.
- I need to acknowledge to myself and the other person that I do not understand the information being given.

**How will this learning be applied in the future?**

- I will ensure that I have a good understanding of what the module entails and how the assessment relates to the learning outcomes.
- I will address my feelings associated with asking for help and further explanation.
- I will tell students if I am new to teaching a module and work with them in less formal ways.

As indicated earlier, a registered nurse is also expected to keep a portfolio of evidence to demonstrate learning for the NMC. A reflective journal is a good starting point to demonstrate what and how you are learning. How you interact with different people is also important, because nursing is about communicating with a variety of different people. Group dynamics are often key to learning and need to be given early attention (Watson, 2024). Activity 9.8 will help you get started with logging such experiences.

## Activity 9.8 Reflection

Think of a recent experience (this could be from within the university or from practice). Now write about the following using one of the models discussed in Chapter 4:

- Describe the experience.
- What essential factors contributed to this experience and are there significant features?
- When you have kept your journal for a week or so, revisit it and consider the following:
- What are the themes emerging from the journal entries?
- What sense do you make of this and using what evidence?

*As this activity is based on your personal experiences, there is an outline answer to only part of this activity at the end of the chapter.*

It is human to want to blame someone else if things do not go according to plan, or if we feel embarrassed by our mistake or oversight. Expressing dissatisfaction with others is known as a form of 'othering' that can remove personal responsibility and accountability to address the situation. It is important, as a professional, to identify and acknowledge when this happens.

If you find yourself starting to use 'othering', there is an option, through reflection, consciously to reject this path (Freshwater, 2000). In this case, reflection and open dialogue are vital, but can be confronting if we are less confident. Writing in the privacy of your reflective journal about your options to deal with the situation is a good starting point for taking proactive action, rather than leaving things to drift and relationships to suffer. The reflective journal is a useful tool for evaluating your strengths, weaknesses, interests and areas for development through reviewing difficult issues and the emerging themes, as discussed at the start of this section. These journal entries can inform your personal development planning and are discussed next.

## Personal development planning

Reflection may create vulnerability in terms of exposing thinking and practice to criticism, and self-concept to realignment (Padykula, 2017; Ruyak et al., 2017). This suggests that reflection and self-awareness take courage, commitment, cognitive insight and emotional resilience. Planning involves reflecting on strengths and areas for improvement, and the interplay between the past and the future, to inform and shape implementation strategies, and translate them into actions. We perhaps need to refocus at this point by reminding ourselves that reflection is a learning strategy, leading to personal and/or professional development. As such, the action that results from such processes requires courage and commitment to try something new, acknowledge the possibility of being wrong, but still recognise the learning gain. This means making use of past learning experiences to interpret present practice and knowledge when writing reflectively, and for personal development planning, projecting outcomes and perhaps further learning into the future. This is an important point to consider when thinking about your learning contracts and whether they are product, rather than process-focused.

A product-focused plan may be dictated by time constraints but may not achieve the ongoing learning process, raising questions of accountability for both practice supervisors and learners. In this regard, feedback is an important component of reviewing progress, in that it provides evaluative information that can be reflected on and incorporated into planning future action and learning. It is important to have thought through what you are attempting to achieve, and your potential commitment, to ensure that you can deliver consistently and equitably on the activities. Table 9.1 gives some headings that you might consider as part of your personal development planning.

As illustrated in Table 9.1, it is important to identify learning objectives that you want to achieve from a situation and ensure that you understand what is expected of you. It is equally important that you articulate your expectations when going into practice, or when being asked to complete independent study. This is helpful for you because it means that: (1) you have clarity in terms of expectations; (2) it is beneficial for your practice or academic supervisor because they are clear as to your level of understanding; and (3) most importantly, you are taking control of your learning by being proactive. Activity 9.9 offers an opportunity to think reflectively about these issues.

*Table 9.1* Headings to organise your personal development

| What are my learning and development needs? | What do I want to gain from this development? | What support do I need and from whom? | Evaluation/review |
|---|---|---|---|
| **Practitioner:** I need to learn more about how to build positive learning relationships. | 1. Be able to support a range of students by creating a positive learning environment. | 1. Organise an experienced practice supervisor who will support and advise me in developing a positive learning environment. | 1. Evaluate whether the student is settled in the clinical environment and whether they feel comfortable and safe on the placement. |
| Learning objective:<br>By week 10 of supporting a student on placement, I am able to:<br>• Demonstrate understanding factors influencing how students integrate into, and learn from, practice settings.<br>• Provide constructive support to allow student transition from one learning environment to another.<br>• Have working relationships to support learning for the entry to register. | 2. Develop awareness of and understand which factors influence my student's learning.<br>3. Develop a plan of action to help the student adapt to a new placement.<br>4. Be confident that I have supported the student to develop professional and interprofessional relationships. | 2. Organise an experienced practice supervisor such as a practice assessor to support and advise me in the assessment process.<br>3. Discuss which skills the student has achieved in previous placements and what they need to achieve in this placement.<br>4. Discuss how the student learns and what they expect from my practice supervision. | 2. Review the student's progress every 3 weeks and establish whether they have sufficient opportunity to achieve their learning objectives.<br>3. Ask the student for specific feedback on my practice supervisor style.<br>4. Final student placement evaluation. |

*(Continued)*

*Table 9.1* (Continued)

| What are my learning and development needs? | What do I want to gain from this development? | What support do I need and from whom? | Evaluation/review |
|---|---|---|---|
| **Student:** I need to learn more about drug administration.<br>Learning objective:<br>By week 10 of my placement, I am able to explain and administer six medications in terms of:<br>• Action<br>• Effect/indication<br>• Route<br>• Dose<br>• Common side effects (in relation to a patient)<br>• Risks (in relation to a patient)<br>• Drug calculation (in relation to a patient)<br>• Correct management, administration and storage of the medication.<br>• Safe administration (in relation to an identified individual patient with specification of the route used). | 1. To be more proficient and have greater knowledge of different drug groups.<br>2. To be aware of, and recognise, risks and side effects of the medications I administer. | 1. My practice supervisor to give me opportunity to practice.<br>2. Access to formulary books.<br>3. Create opportunities to discuss the medications I see in practice, with my practice supervisor, in relation to actual patients. | 1. Review progress with my practice supervisor at the second and third meeting dates.<br>2. Evaluate with my practice supervisor whether I have achieved the learning objectives set at the start of the placement.<br>3. Set learning objectives for my next placement that allow me to develop my skills and knowledge. |

### Activity 9.9 Critical thinking

Think about your next placement, or next year, if appropriate. If you are an experienced practitioner, think about your next appraisal. Now consider the following questions:

- What are your strengths?
- What are your weaknesses?
- How do you know this (are there aspects that make you feel uncertain)?
- What are you planning to do about this?
- What, from reflection, do you need to take forward (what opportunities will this offer)?

Now write a reflective account to draw these strengths, weaknesses, opportunities and threats (SWOT) into a whole as evidence for your portfolio.

*As this activity is based on your personal experiences, there is an outline answer to only part of this activity at the end of the chapter.*

Personal development planning is a way to develop agency and take control of your learning and ensure that it is linked to your needs. This principle continues throughout your career and often a personal learning plan forms the basis of annual appraisal meetings. For registered healthcare professionals, it is incorporated into professional validation and triennial reviews.

Providing evidence of your personal development requires you to write about it within formal assignments, whether as a preregistration learner or an experienced practitioner undertaking further study. This leads us to consider reflective writing in assignments.

## Reflective writing in assignments

When discussing reflective writing it is worth considering an interesting point made by Hargreaves (2004, p. 200), suggesting that we generally produce three types of reflective narrative:

- *valedictory*: where we save a 'bad situation' and come out victorious at the end;
- *condemnatory*: where a situation goes wrong and we cannot resolve it, and emerge feeling dissatisfied and, possibly, guilty;
- *redemptive*: where we respond inappropriately to a situation, but then redeem ourselves, suggesting that we have improved our practice.

These three narrative types may develop unconsciously, and it is worth trying to recognise whether you favour a particular approach as we discuss reflective writing in assignments.

Nursing's voice is situated in practice and practitioners 'know nursing' as insiders. When including reflective accounts in academic work, we sometimes do not include threatening or contentious experiences or oversimplify into more acceptable versions to meet course requirements, rather than using the opportunity to make sense of the experience. For example, we might not write about mistakes or less positive placement experiences for fear of being penalised. In this respect we need to remain mindful that there is an ethical tension if unsafe or unprofessional practice situations are included in reflective accounts because academic staff are also professionally bound to escalate concerns while balancing confidentiality with the duty of care to the learner. There is normally an escalation policy that is clear to all parties, with well-defined outcomes for the process. Within this, academic and practice responsibility is shared to enable learning and build your self-confidence. Clearly, this can happen only in an open and trusting environment that calls for clear intercollegiate communication and sound professional values from all parties concerned. This shared responsibility to maintain professional values is strengthened by the understanding practitioners have of the process and cyclical nature of healthcare, the contextual decision-making and educational practice making this 'inside knowledge' easier to articulate. The complementary, academic, voice in nursing sometimes feels less straightforward, requiring intellectual effort to negotiate different viewpoints, parameters and theoretical models, but the combination represents the professional voice of nursing.

Reflection, as already discussed, is a valuable tool to learning and teaching, but must be purposeful and carefully integrated within curricula to achieve relevant and credible learning. Marking and, therefore, producing reflective writing in assignments are focused on the breadth and depth of the reflective content. This follows a continuum of whether written reflections are perceptive and significant with convincing conclusions, or whether they are superficial and lack relevance. Developing our reflective writing means moving beyond a description of reflection and the immediate context of the situation to offering perceptive insights and that includes subtle thought and originality. This can be achieved by:

- considering what theoretical concepts are active in the situation;
- any unique features that the situation is demonstrating;
- what your view is, based on experience and reflection – give examples;
- keeping the focus on *your* practice and not generalising to some abstract generic view.

Below is a brief example of a paragraph that might be part of reflective writing in assignments.

### Example of reflective writing in assignments

The long-term conditions module is making me consider how I approach and think about people with long-term and often complex illnesses. I realise that I am often focused on the tasks within the context of providing their specific care and forget about the patient's experience and expertise. It is easy to get caught up in problem-solving and leave them out. I find that I do not include the patient in the decision-making because I do not want to give the impression that I am uncertain or lack knowledge and skill in a particular area. I try to integrate the theory I have learnt in my practice, but I am aware that trying to think theoretically separates me from subjective and intuitive elements. I am afraid that my care can become objectified rather than me responding to the person. I know that I need to communicate my decision-making to the patient so that they are included and can offer their insights and expert experience from living with their condition and, consequently, be part of the solution. I will revisit person-centred care, shared decision-making and partnership literature, and make a conscious effort to include patients in my assessment and decision-making. I will discuss my plan of action with my practice supervisor and ask that they observe me with patients and provide me with specific feedback.

It can be helpful to analyse reflection more deeply through guided reflection, as discussed in Chapter 8. When you are involved in guided reflection it is important to record the learning that this generates, to ensure that it is captured. We now consider how this is another form of reflective writing.

## Recording guided reflection

Guided reflection can help address some of the ethical issues identified earlier around student vulnerability. This is achieved by using a partnership approach between student and practice/academic supervisor, to set clear outcomes for the issue and provide support during the process. The issue of a reconstructed past remains challenging, although careful questioning of and attentive listening to yourself, as well as questioning and active listening by the reflective guide, may facilitate this. You may find it helpful to use the template (based on the one provided in Chapter 1) to record guided reflection.

- Pro forma for documenting guided reflection.
    - Practice-based experience:
    - Main points identified from reflection on the experience:
    - Main points identified from guided exploration of the experience:
    - Learning points:
    - How will this learning be applied in practice?
    - Professional development achieved?

## Chapter summary

Reflection often dissolves in the reality of everyday work and life. Holism is achieved by embedding a continuous cycle of experimentation and review through reflective writing. Reflection is an art that requires insight and self-awareness, and it will take longer than the time allocated for a programme to develop fully because it is an aspect of professional life-long learning. Writing is one way to start embedding the process. The activities in this chapter have provided different opportunities to expand your writing and develop different techniques that could generate further reflective insights.

## Brief outline answers

In this section, answers to the chapter's activities will be outlined and explained.

### Activity 9.1 Reflection

Reflecting on Molly Case's poem 'Nursing the Nation', you may have responded in different ways. For example:

- Emotional: the content of Molly Case's poem may have resonated strongly with your own experiences or, perhaps, you were struck by the power of the words and their intonation.
- Sad: the poem's content may have conjured up memories of working in extreme conditions during the COVID-19 pandemic and the contradiction of your work as a nurse with laconic public and political attitudes.
- Irritated: perhaps you found the presentation of the poem altogether too melodramatic and patronising.

The important part of this exercise is to reflect on your reaction to the poem and try to analyse what triggered your response and why you responded as you did. What does this say about you? Do you recognise your response to service users and carers or colleagues and peers? Does your response impact positively/negatively on your care and/or collegiality?

### Activity 9.2 Reflection

Joe focuses on emotions and the impact on his learning. He has thought of what Ross could do differently and how he might respond if he were a practice supervisor.

Ross considers his and Joe's feelings. He has considered how his actions contributed to the current situation and what he can do about it.

Joe and Ross have considered a communication book, but neither has reflected on addressing the emotional aspects. Further analysis could add depth to the reflection and include how the actions and influence of others and events could influence future behaviour.

Things that you may have thought about in terms of how Joe and Ross could develop their reflection further include:

- Joe could explore why he feels bullied and victimised by the situation. Where does this come from (his biography)? What risks are involved in maintaining this behaviour? Could this (rather than Ross) be limiting his development on the ward? Does he understand how the lack of communication could be seen as unprofessional and what it means for the organisation and operationalisation of care? Which learning objectives could Joe formulate to overcome this feeling? How could Joe apply feedback guidelines to the situation? What would be the aim of a meeting with Ross?

- Ross could reflect on several issues; for example, his strategies for coping with stress and how he sets his boundaries. Why did he accept responsibility for three students and team leadership when he has little experience? Another area could be his impatience and his perfectionism. A third area might be his communication strategy as practice supervisor and role model – issues about emotional intelligence and power could inform his reflection in this area.

## Activity 9.3 Reflection

- Faheed might sense tensions within the group and who the leaders of the group are. He might recognise with whom he should discuss the group dynamics to achieve the best outcome. This could indicate his leadership potential.
- Faheed might have learnt about his communication and assertiveness skills by how his interaction had inspired the group. This could increase his confidence.
- He might have identified how to minimise barriers between different professions. Faheed's story might have said something like:
    - My uncle was injured in an accident. He was ventilated for 4 days in intensive care and then transferred to a ward. He was discharged 3 weeks later but needed help at home for another 2 weeks. The professionals involved in his recovery included doctors, nurses, physiotherapists, occupational therapists and community nurses. I saw the different professions working closely together in the intensive care unit, each demonstrating their expertise. The professionals consulted each other on an equal level as they worked within their own professional boundaries.
    - On the ward there was less joined-up communication, and different professions worked independently. I reflected on this. Intensive care focuses on acute detail and the professionals contribute to understanding the case. On the ward, patients may be at different stages of recovery and have diverse needs. The opportunities to collaborate and interact can be disjointed, resulting in a task-based approach, so it can be difficult to construct a picture of each profession's contribution to holistic care.
    - Through this experience I recognise that physiotherapists help with physical mobility rehabilitation and are vital in preventing chest infections by clearing the chest of secretions. Occupational therapists ensure that people are ready to manage independently at home. Doctors and nurses' roles overlap in that the doctors prescribe treatment based on nurses' observations. I think that interprofessional collaboration is based on professionals recognising each other's strengths and expertise and avoiding power issues.

## Activity 9.4 Reflection

The articles required for this activity are:

- **Aydogdu, A.L.F. & Disbudak, B.** (2025). Interpersonal conflicts in nursing through the lens of senior nursing students: A qualitative study. *Nurse Education Today*, 144. https://doi.org/10.1016/j.nedt.2024.106398.
- **Freshwater, D.** (2000). Crosscurrents against cultural narration in nursing. *Journal of Advanced Nursing, 32*(2), 481–484.
- **Hutchinson, M., Vickers, M., Jackson, D. & Wilkes, L.** (2006). Workplace bullying in nursing: Towards a more critical organisational perspective. *Nursing Inquiry, 13*(2), 118–126.

## Activity 9.6 Reflection

Mia broke corporate confidentiality by naming the healthcare **trust** she worked in and the institution where she was studying. This meant that her work could, potentially, identify where any situation she was talking about was located. Some people call this the 'on the bus test'. If she left the work in a public place by mistake, are there sufficient identifiers to locate where situations are happening? In terms of the consequences of breaching confidentiality, for Mia these would be greater (although these still depend on the seriousness of the breach), because she is a registered nurse and therefore accountable for her actions. The consequences for Josh, as a student, if he had followed the same actions as Mia, are less serious (although these still depend on the seriousness of the breach), because he has a responsibility for maintaining confidentiality, but is not yet a registered accountable practitioner. The best option is to leave any identifiers out of any account.

## Activity 9.7 Reflection

Although the content and structure of your reflection are likely to be unique to you, there are some common rules you may have followed. You may have plotted the reflective story as a sequence of scenes. Or perhaps you have chosen specific music, if using dance. If using poetry, you may have considered whether to use a chorus or rhyming mechanism to emphasise particular points. All of these considerations are important. When writing creatively, it is important to take a few things into account:

- Use a quiet, comfortable location, free from distraction and where you feel safe to write without anxiety that you may be interrupted or questioned.
- Organise your thoughts, ideas and/or emotions. It may help you to organise your thoughts by constructing a mind map that expresses your ideas (Figure 9.1).
- Read your work, slowly and aloud. Then edit it to include extra or different punctuation, change terminology or language, possibly change the style from a passive to an active sentence construction, establish whether it should be in the present, past or future tense, etc.
- Leave your work to rest for a few days and then reread it in the same way again and decide what (if anything) needs changing. You will know when it is ready.

## Activity 9.8 Reflection

The themes you identified may have been concerned with communication skills, decision-making and relationships with service users, carers, peers, practice colleagues, clients, or lecturers.

## Activity 9.9 Critical thinking

You might identify strengths in relation to particular skills and others that you want to improve. Possibly confidence or assertiveness have featured as an area for improvement – you may know this from previous feedback and your own reflections. Or perhaps you need more knowledge or practical skills. As a registered nurse this might involve a study day or training, which you need to request from your line manager. These insights should inform your learning contract; you will find that your reflection after planning your personal development is likely to be more positive because you will have developed some agency and taken control of your learning and development. (For a discussion on agency, return to Chapter 3.)

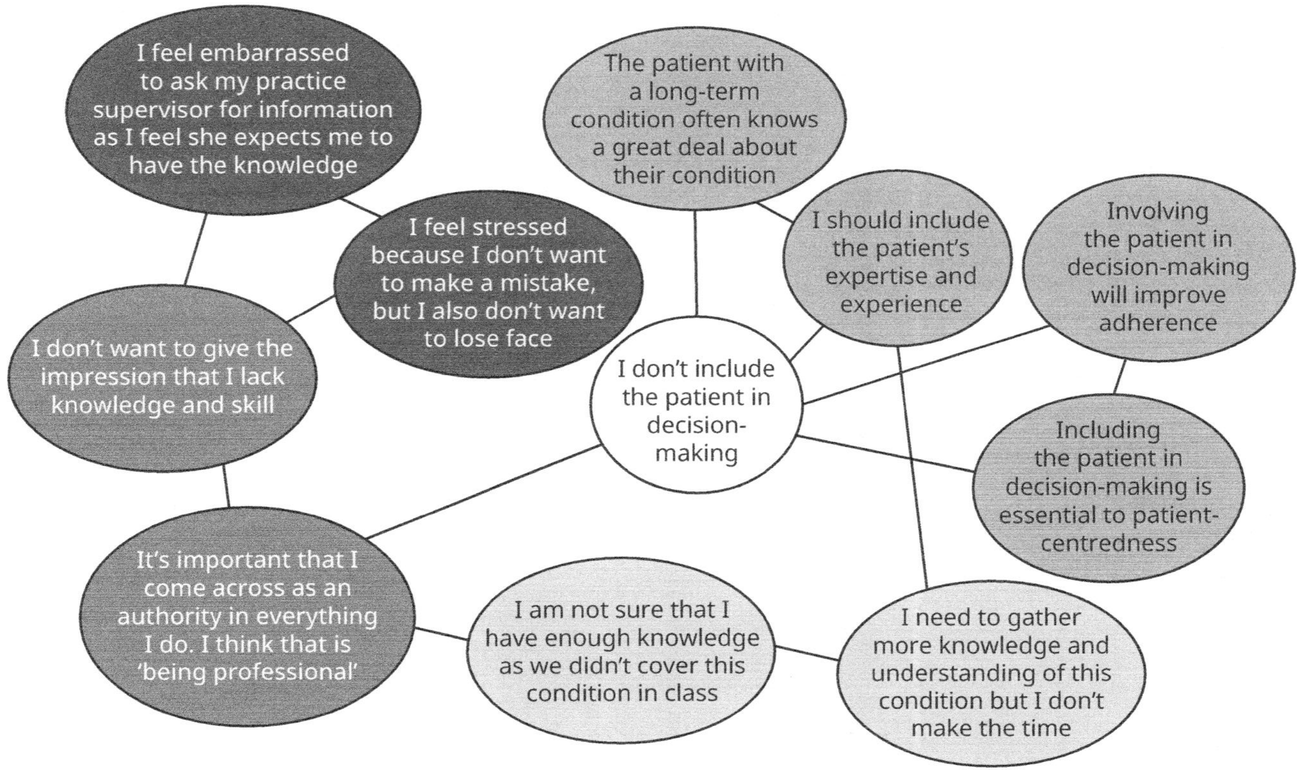


*Figure 9.1* Mind map example to organise your thoughts and ideas

## Further reading

**Bolton, G. & Delderfield, R.** (2018). *Reflective practice: Writing and professional development* (5th ed.). Sage.

An in-depth guide to reflective writing, which is beyond the scope of this chapter.

**Mahon, P. & O'Neill, M.** (2020). Through the looking glass: The rabbit hole of reflective practice. *British Journal of Nursing*, 29(13), 777–783.

This is an interesting and critical discussion of reflection.

**Price, B.** (2024). *Critical thinking and writing for nursing students* (6th ed.). Sage.

This book provides a good explanation and examples of how to write reflective essays applying critical thinking skills that map to the NMC's *Future Nurse: Standards of Proficiency for Registered Nurses* (NMC, 2018a).

## Useful websites

**www.nmc.org.uk/globalassets/sitedocuments/revalidation/completed-revalidation-forms-and-templates.pdf**

Registered nurses should view this chapter as complementary to information included on the NMC website (and consider the learning activities in terms of the reflective accounts required for revalidation).

**www.youtube.com/watch?v=JHue5ZQf9jY**

YouTube clip 'Nursing the Nation', a poem by student nurse Molly Case from the 2013 Royal College of Nursing Congress.

# Chapter 10 Using new media for reflecting

## NMC Future Nurse: Standards of Proficiency for Registered Nurses

This chapter will address the following platforms and proficiencies:

**Platform 1: Being an accountable professional**

1.11 Communicate effectively using a range of skills and strategies with colleagues and people at all stages of life and with a range of mental, physical, cognitive and behavioural health challenges.

1.17 Take responsibility for continuous self-reflection, seeking and responding to support and feedback to develop their professional knowledge and skills.

## Chapter aims

After reading this chapter, you will be able to:

- identify different types of media that can be used for reflection;
- assess the advantages and avoid the pitfalls of using media for reflection;
- develop a reflective script for a media narrative;
- identify how you can contribute to others' reflective learning.

## Case Study 10.1: Sonia's reflective experience

Sonia has just started her children's nursing programme. One of the first tasks she has to do is to set up her electronic portfolio using different pages for different parts of her learning experience. She is concerned about completing this task because she has not used an e-portfolio tool before. However, after an introductory

*(Continued)*

(Continued)

talk about how to get started from her course tutor, Julie, Sonia manages to set up her e-portfolio with named pages for her skills, personal development planning with actions, reflective diary and practice development.

Sonia starts to use her reflective journal to log her learning experiences of lectures. She mentions her clinical science tutor by name, saying how impressed she is with the resources he provides to the class. After sharing her e-portfolio for feedback on her writing, Julie comments that confidentiality needs to be maintained by not including people's names and that Sonia is ready to reflect on these experiences. Sonia goes back to her reflective journal and edits out the clinical science tutor's name and thinks about the 'so what' of her experience.

When Sonia starts her first placement, she is excited and decides that it would be helpful for her learning to reflect on her experiences. Each week she writes a reflective log about what she has learnt in placement.

Remembering Julie's comment about maintaining confidentiality, Sonia ensures that she does not name any people, the placement or the organisation where it is located. Just before returning to university and submitting her e-portfolio, Sonia reflects on the sum total of her practice experiences by considering the question 'so what?' Julie places a further comment on Sonia's e-portfolio practice page affirming Sonia's reflective ability and her progression and learning from the feedback that she receives.

### Activity 10.1 Reflection

- Using your knowledge of reflection from your reading so far, make a list of the characteristics of any of the media tools mentioned above that would help you to reflect and why.
- In what ways do you think you might use the different media mentioned to reflect?
- Are there any other media, not mentioned, that you could use?

*This activity is based on your experience; however, there is a set of questions at the end of the chapter to assist you with this learning activity.*

## Introduction

As technology progresses, new media become available, and opportunities increase for creative ways of reflecting. It is, therefore, important that we are familiar with the options available, to ensure that we use what is available and that we engage with, and teach, others.

Using e-technology in different ways helps you prepare for the ongoing electronic record changes and developments in practice. However, as highlighted in Case Study 10.1, media also pose potential problems that you need to guard against to protect those in your care and avoid misconduct resulting from not adhering to *The Code* (NMC, 2018b). Confidentiality has always been an issue, but the use of media and the inability specifically to control information once it has been posted electronically (rather than using paper-based documentation) can result in unintended confidentiality breaches.

This chapter introduces some of the media that you might use in your reflective learning. It also highlights the opportunities and dangers posed by such media and identifies ways that you can use media responsibly and professionally. The chapter offers you an opportunity to develop a reflective script and concludes with how to translate this into a digital story.

## Different types of media

Media refers to technology and virtual platforms that make connecting with others much easier. Virtual communication is continually developing and the list of examples given below is clearly incomplete, but some of these technological tools are:

- social networking, such as Facebook, YouTube, Instagram, etc.;
- instant messaging, such as WhatsApp, Snapchat, WeChat, X, Skype, Facebook Messenger, texting, etc.;
- email;
- creative digital media; for example, image-sharing software, such as Movavi Video Editor Plus, Audacity, TikTok, YouTube Vlog, etc.

Greenwood (2011) provides an interesting commentary on Ohler's (2008) work in which they used the term 'new media' because it allowed for expansion and change in an evolving medium that remains relevant. Stein et al. (2020) and Lee (2020) explore the medium of virtual technology in more depth, highlighting the challenges associated with parasocial communication and authenticity; these considerations will be discussed in relation to reflection later in the chapter.

As Case Study 10.1 highlights, media offer different possibilities for reflection. One example is the e-portfolio, which offers structure by providing templates to guide your writing and the opportunity to collect feedback when they are shared. The information can be kept private within the virtual learning environment or shared with others whom you invite and send a link that allows them to access your work. Feedback is given via a comment section. This system has advantages for the student, practice supervisor and personal tutor as, once all parties have been invited, they can follow your progress and provide communication and feedback in real time.

Your portfolio should include a section of reflective learning because this is a key aspect of *The Code* (NMC, 2018b) in terms of keeping your knowledge up to date. The Nursing and Midwifery Council (NMC) expects all nurses to keep a portfolio and can call on this evidence at the point of registration and beyond (NMC, 2017). (See also *Successful Professional Portfolios for Nursing Students* (Reed, 2015) in this series).

Social networking is useful for sharing ideas as it enables discussion of issues, sharing learning and following key experts through blogs and vlogs. However, virtual media, especially open sites such as Facebook, Instagram, X and TikTok, need to be used with caution, as discussed later in this chapter.

Creative media allow you to upload images and audio to create videos or digital stories, offering the potential for more creative reflection. Examples of free downloadable media programs that enable you to do this include Movavi Video Editor Plus, Audacity and YouTube Vlog, among others. These can be used to create media files from the images, sounds and narration that you input. It is important to maintain confidentiality from a different perspective when doing this because images can provide recognition of location and settings. It is essential to remain mindful that this consideration also applies to images of the university setting, clinical skills suite, simulation laboratories, etc. As highlighted by Lee (2020), authenticity is an important aspect to be considered as the anonymity of virtual communication and virtual reality can result in our boundaries blurring and can allow us to take on whichever persona we like. Stein et al. (2020) discuss this in more detail, addressing the challenges of parasocial interaction and parasocial relationships in which we engage with the image of an individual and their ideas via virtual reality using the communication strategies we have developed in face-to-face communication. This can result in us accepting all that is said as 'truth' without the nuances of further interrogation which would normally occur. The 'warning' highlighted by Lee (2020) becomes tangible as the person delivering the virtual message may not be who they say they are, clouding our criticality. Similarly, when we work with a reflective blog or vlog, producing virtual reality in anonymity and isolation calls for our integrity to maintain confidentiality and remain true to ourselves as individuals and professionals (O'Connor et al., 2022).

> *The NMC (2025) reminds us to "Use all forms of spoken, written and digital communication (including social media and networking sites) responsibly." (The Code, paragraph 20.10)*

As an alternative, you could use the narrated PowerPoint option in association with copyright-free images to create a video file using a Windows app. This approach can harness different thought processes; for example, you might choose an image as a metaphor for what would require many words to explain. Viewers make sense of the meaning framed by their own biographical experience (for more information on this, revisit Chapter 3). Creating stories requires discipline, structure, scripting, critical analysis and editing, which are also the skills needed for critical reflection. See Activity 10.1 to reconsider how you might use a variety of media.

On completion of the activity, you may have considered how different forms of media allow you to express yourself differently in ways that are not yet fully formed. Or you may have thought about how media could enable you to interact with others to get feedback on your ideas to develop your reflective thinking and experience. Although interaction can be an advantage, you need to be aware of some pitfalls.

## Advantages and pitfalls of new media

Media, as suggested, can enable dynamic articulation of reflections. This includes synchronous approaches such as social networking as well as asynchronous methods such as discussion boards, blogs and vlogs. The advantages of these are that they bring nurses together in new ways and are not limited to locations, providing opportunities for development and giving nurses an international platform to discuss issues and sharing good practice (NMC 2025; O'Connor et al., 2022). For example, through talking to nurses from other countries, we can compare and contrast different healthcare systems across the world and reflect on our own role at the same time. New media offer opportunities to study at a distance and to keep in contact with developing ideas without having to sit in a classroom with others. This makes education programmes more accessible to a wider variety of people and provides opportunities for group work that would otherwise not be possible.

There are, however, also inherent risks. The Royal College of Nursing (RCN, 2023) highlights that once information has been shared on social media it is out there forever, everything previously shared can be found. Recognising that nurses use social networking sites, the NMC (2025), Jones (2019), and RCN (2019) produced guidance and advice, noting that nurses and midwives can put their registration at risk and students may jeopardise their ability to join the register if they:

- share confidential information online;
- post inappropriate comments about staff or patients;
- use social networking sites to bully and intimidate colleagues;
- pursue personal relationships with patients and service users;
- distribute sexually explicit material;
- use social networking sites in a way that is unlawful.

The NMC (2025) advises that conduct in the real world and online should be viewed as one and the same, and conduct should always be in keeping with the standards of *The Code* (NMC, 2018b). Now consider Case Study 10.2 and answer the questions in Activity 10.2, later in this chapter.

### Case Study 10.2: Stacey's image-sharing experience

Stacey is a newly qualified learning disability nurse. During her preparation programme Stacey kept in touch with her peers and university life via Facebook. Once

*(Continued)*

(Continued)

qualified, she updated her profile to reflect this. Stacey enjoys travelling and is a keen photographer. She enjoys sharing her images with her friends and usually uses Facebook to do so. She recently uploaded some holiday images of Indigenous Australians to Facebook and added some comments. Stacey is surprised when she is called to see her manager because a complaint has been made about how she represents the equality and diversity policy of the organisation on social media.

Remember, our interpretation of images is subjective and can result in unintended consequences and Stacey would have had very different ideas about the purpose of her images to those of other viewers. The fact that she has listed her occupation on her profile may further influence viewers' ideas about what she might be trying to say through posting her images. The narrative of images is a strong focus of media offering creative potential but, as Stacey's experience highlights, there are also responsibilities to consider.

In 2009, the RCN produced legal advice on using the internet. This emphasises the importance of reading and adhering to the information technology (IT) policy of the organisation you are in and ensuring that you uphold the reputation of both your profession and the organisation. For the qualified practitioner, this means ensuring that personal behaviour does not compromise professional standing. For the student nurse this would mean familiarising yourself with, and adhering to, NMC professional guidelines, the IT policy of the educational organisation responsible for your programme and the healthcare trusts in which your placements are located.

Additionally, in 2025 the NMC produced guidance on using social media responsibly that provides clear direction for professional and private use in line with the Code for nursing and midwifery professions.

Most of this is straightforward advice to follow, but there are times when boundaries blur and it can be difficult to remember who you are professionally. Consider Case Study 10.3 and complete Activity 10.2 to clarify what you think you would do.

### Case Study 10.3: Alistair's social networking experience

Alistair is a year three adult nurse trainee on placement at a general practice (GP) surgery. He enjoyed this placement because of the diversity of the work and the people with whom he came into contact. He became very friendly with his practice supervisor, Colin. Alistair asked Colin if he would be interested in becoming a friend on his social networking site. Colin agreed and told Alistair to send him an invitation. That evening Alistair was on the site and sent Colin an invitation to become a friend. In his invitation Alistair said that he very much enjoyed working with Colin at the GP surgery. Colin accepted the invitation and he and Alistair have been swapping messages about their interests outside work. There are some issues that Alistair wants to learn more about in relation to his placement, but he does not discuss these on the social networking site because this would not be appropriate. He catches up with Colin at work about them instead. At the end of his placement Alistair asks Colin to keep in touch, which he agrees to do.

### Activity 10.2 Reflection

After reading Case Study 10.2 about Stacey's experience and Case Study 10.3 about Alistair and Colin, answer the following questions:

- What should Stacey have thought about before uploading her photos and comments?
- What are the main issues in the case study concerning Alistair and Colin?
- What might be the outcomes for Stacey, Alistair, and Colin?
- What might you do differently?

*There are outline answers to these questions at the end of the chapter.*

Activity 10.2 has given you the opportunity to think about some of the challenges involved in separating professional and private life, and keeping appropriate boundaries, particularly when you feel that people are friends. Reflecting on such experiences is important for developing and maintaining professional behaviour. Your professional integrity is essential to becoming registered or keeping your registration if you are a registered practitioner. We continue to consider positive ways in which media can be used for reflection by exploring how to develop stories.

# Developing a reflective story using new media

Storytelling has been a traditional part of human communication for centuries and stories are a useful tool for developing understanding. It is a powerful means for developing knowledge and ***self-reliance*** in your nursing practice (Beck & Neil, 2021; Lee & Suh, 2025). Considering a significant issue and creating the story that surrounds it helps to clarify your thinking and reasoning, and to reflect differently than is possible in a written assignment (Moore, 2023).

Developing reflective stories using new media enables you to:

- organise deep reflection, review, analyse, and order information (e.g. a project, a topic, an experience);
- value emotional/personal input; "Honestly, you can bring home so many points with a story."

- make sense of experiences.
- encourage cooperative activity: "After receiving permission from the student who had created the digital story, the instructor used this same digital story to make a point"
- create powerful end-products that can have a transformative effect on maker and viewer alike; "Talking about creating digital stories, student–created videos engage more than anything else."
- develop capacity for self-review;
- build skills such as confidence, empathy, self-care. "I think that [digital stories] help students feel more like what it's like to be in that position. It can promote empathy".

(Beck & Neil, 2021)

## Case Study 10.4: Person-centred care

'Where's Mike?' asked the gruff visitor, Ben, at the desk. Maggie glanced at Stella nervously. 'Room 9', she calmly replied. Ben walked up the corridor and disappeared into Mike's room. Mike had been transferred to the limb surgery unit following a motorcycle accident. He had been filtering to go off a roundabout and had been crushed by a lorry. His lower leg was damaged beyond repair and had to be amputated. Mike was struggling to come to terms with his injury, often becoming angry and resentful.

This is Maggie's first qualified nurse post, and she is still getting used to it. She is learning how to dress stump wounds and bandage them correctly. What Maggie is finding harder, though, is learning how to connect with the wounded person. She comes from a background where people are valued as individuals, and she wants to apply those values to nursing. The problem is, how does she work with Mike in a way that is meaningful for him and values his individuality?

They start to chat. Mike says that he finds being admitted on the limb surgery unit boring because there is nothing for him to do. Maggie asks him what he normally does. He says that he works on art designs for motorcycles. He has a website where he showcases his work, and people contact him, or they approach him at the events he attends. He does not want to miss the motorcycle show at the end of the month. He is worried that his business will suffer. Maggie calls Ben on the phone and asks him to bring Mike's laptop and also calls the occupational therapist and asks her to source some art materials for Mike. Mike starts to use these to create design ideas and appears more purposeful. Maggie also talks to the physiotherapist about his objective of getting to the motorcycle show. The physiotherapist tailors Mike's exercise regime to include walking on uneven terrain.

At the end of the month Mike's friend Ben, who is less abrasive now the staff have come to know him better, takes Mike to the motorcycle show. Maggie thinks she will ask Mike if he is willing to share his experiences and recovery with others as they often treat bikers on the unit.

The process of creating the story makes it an embodied experience, which allows you to visualise and relive the situation, and it is important for deepening your understanding and learning. 'Embodiment' means that the experience is lived and owned by you as the person reflecting, and unconscious aspects are brought to light. Our experiences are informed by the *appearance, disappearance and reappearance of events and people making our world seem familiar* (Horsdal, 2012, p. 10). However, we cannot perceive these influences unless we can see the whole story.

## Case Study 10.5: Naeve's critical incident experience

Naeve was working in a mental health secure unit placement. She was in the third year of her mental health nursing programme and was due to qualify in 3 months. She had finished a stretch of duties and, on one of her days off, decided to reflect on a particular issue that had given her work satisfaction. The unit had some patients with complex problems. One of these was Jeff, who had been sectioned and admitted after smashing up the family home and having an altercation with the police. He had been signed off work with severe stress preceding this event. His family had found the experience extremely traumatic and were reluctant to visit him. He had a sister who lived 2 hours' travelling time away. Naeve could see that Jeff was withdrawn and did not speak much. Each day that she was on shift she spent some time sitting with him, trying to draw him out. By the second week he was starting to mumble some responses. By the third week Naeve managed to coax Jeff to come downstairs for his lunch. His sister had been enquiring after Jeff regularly. In that third week Naeve asked Jeff if he wanted to see his sister and he agreed. Jeff asked for Naeve to be present when they met.

Jeff's sister Miriam met him in the common room. At first everything appeared to be going well, but then Jeff lost his temper when Miriam asked him where he would go on leaving the unit because he could not go back home. Naeve helped Miriam leave the room and returned to Jeff. Although she felt anxious, Naeve was able to maintain a calm exterior, which gradually helped Jeff relax. Naeve's practice supervisor, Andrew, had been observing her communication skills during this interaction and was very impressed with Naeve's handling of this volatile situation. Andrew gave Naeve a glowing report before she left the placement.

Naeve used a private blog to reflect on the incident and her overall feelings about the placement over the last few weeks. She felt she had made some real progress in her interaction with Jeff. She found this satisfying because it appeared to affirm her communication ability. When Jeff had become agitated and angry in his interaction with his sister, Naeve had reacted quickly to remove Miriam from danger and calm the situation, despite feeling fearful. She knew that this was part of what she would need to do as a mental health nurse and was pleased that the way in which she had managed the critical incident had been affirmed by her practice supervisor.

*(Continued)*

(Continued)

When she considered what she might have done differently she thought about whether she should have called for help or sent Miriam to get help when she left the room. The reason she had not done this was because she felt confident in her own abilities and the therapeutic relationship she had established with Jeff. Naeve thought that the worst that could have happened was that Jeff might have struck her, but as she had had training in breakaway techniques, she felt able to take care of herself, and preferred to use communication to resolve the situation. The incident had increased her confidence in being able to manage different situations effectively and she felt more prepared for qualifying in the next few months.

## Activity 10.3 Reflection

- Develop a story about the incident described in Case Study 10.3 and Naeve's reflection on it.
- Now try to write a story for a critical incident you have experienced and your reflection on it.

*There is an outline answer to part of this activity at the end of the chapter.*

Writing an event using storytelling helps you to deconstruct and examine different elements before reassembling them in a cohesive whole. Storytelling normally starts with a significant event that engages the reader's attention from the start and has an unfolding plot that connects different aspects in a whole. This requires critical awareness in knowing what to select and what to leave out and how to substantiate important points. The writing should be approximately 200–300 words in length (Matthews-DeNatale, 2013). As stated by Beck and Neil (2021) the skills involved in creating a story using new media include:

- narrative generation;
- reflection;
- analysis of material;
- analysis of self in relation to material;
- organising and sorting information for use;
- use of personal and technological/technical skills.

The first step is to match the script with appropriate images. To do this you will need to access the software that you intend to use and create a storyboard (this can be a series of boxes that link the plot of the script with numbered images). This allows you to place your chosen images on an editing line similar to a film strip. Images can be sourced from your own photographs, from photo-share sites such as **www.flickr.com** and from hand drawings. It is important to make sure that you check and follow copyright rules for any shared images and that you gain consent for any personal photos involving other people.

The next step is to convert the script into an audio file using an appropriate audio editing tool. An example is Audacity, which records you narrating the script. Or, if you are planning to use PowerPoint, you could use the recording element to narrate to PowerPoint. Try to do this in as natural a way as possible in a quiet space, as if you were talking to someone. If you are using PowerPoint, make sure that you wait for any transitions to have completed to avoid words being cut off. This is the first step to converting the script into a digital story.

Once you have matched your audio with the images, you can add titles and save your project. At this stage you should still be able to edit it. You are now ready to review your project file and reflect on whether the story portrays what you intended. It is also helpful at this stage to get other people's feedback, because then you can make editing changes before completing the final story package. Complete Activity 10.4 to see what you can produce.

### Activity 10.4 Reflection

(Note: You will need a headset with a microphone for this activity.)

Download Movavi Video Editor Plus from **www.movavi.com/download-videoeditorplus** on to your computer:

- Find a photo that holds a special meaning for you.
- Think about the memories that are triggered by the photo and write a story about these using the guidance previously given.
- Translate this script into a digital story using the new media software and following the prompts, as suggested above.
- Review your digital story and the processes used to create it and reflect on what you have learnt.

*As this activity is based on your own experiences, there is no outline answer at the end of the chapter.*

We now proceed to explore how sharing stories that have been created using media can contribute to the reflective learning of others.

## Contributing to the reflective learning of others

Sharing your development of the digital story with peers and teachers helps you to improve the quality of the final product but also contributes to the reflective learning of others as they explore the meaning that they make from viewing your story. It is therefore useful to share your practice with others to collaborate in reflecting. As technology progresses, more advanced media are increasingly being used within nursing programmes to bring the service user voice to the fore and to develop learning in more engaging ways. Examples that are used can be found on the Patient Voices website at **www.patientvoices.org.uk**. It is interesting to view different stories and share your reflections on them.

## Chapter summary

This chapter has explored how to use media to develop reflection in different ways. Some of the advantages and pitfalls have been highlighted to help you use these new opportunities constructively, and guard against creating problems for yourself that could affect you professionally and jeopardise your registration. The activities have offered you opportunities to develop your own digital story to reflect on. In the process you will have developed and practised media skills that you can take forward in your own learning and that you can use to contribute to the reflections of others.

## Brief outline answers

In this section, answers to the chapter's activities will be outlined and explained.

### Activity 10.1 Reflection

Although this is not an exhaustive list, you might consider the following elements:

- Are you familiar with the e-portfolio – the aim of the e-portfolio, how it works, how it is structured, what needs to be saved where and so on? Or do you need to revisit the guidance and handbook or access advice from someone in authority?
- Does the e-portfolio have an inbuilt structure, based on a reflective model as discussed in Chapter 4? Or do you have the freedom to use different reflective models?
- How are you able to use the e-portfolio to support your learning, rather than seeing it as a tick-box activity? For example, are you able to identify the learning outcomes for each activity? How do you use the learning outcomes to structure the activity? Are you able to identify and formulate specific areas for your personal and professional development?
- How do you decide what to include and what to leave out of your reflective work? For example, how do you manage confidentiality?
- How do you use the e-portfolio? For example, you could use it to jot points down as they happen and then look back at them over a period of time, or you might set aside a set period of time after each shift or block of shifts, or after specific learning activities.
- Now consider other ways that stimulate you to reflect; perhaps a photograph or picture as a symbol to stimulate your reflection, or a poem that you have read, a film, or music you might associate with a specific situation, service user or family member.

### Activity 10.2 Reflection

The main issues that arise in Case Study 10.2 are:

- Stacey has identified that she is a qualified children's nurse and therefore she is accountable for her actions.
- She is not properly adhering to her organisation's equality and diversity policy or the NMC's Code.

In Case Study 10.3, involving Alistair and Colin, issues arise through:

- the blurring of Alistair's and Colin's professional and private lives, as evidenced in their social networking communication;
- Alistair's mention in his invitation that they both work in a GP surgery.

The potential outcomes for Stacey are that she may receive a warning, which will be kept on her file because she is accountable for her actions. For Alistair, any feedback that Colin gives him as his practice supervisor may be viewed through the lens of social networking and, potentially, not be taken seriously. Possible outcomes for Colin are that he is accountable for his actions and could be putting his registration at risk. By blurring the boundary between his professional role as practice supervisor and communicating socially with Alistair online, Colin cannot guarantee what Alistair might say. Other people could access the posts and that could have professional repercussions. As a student, you might think that it is innocent to develop a friendship with someone. However, as a practice supervisor or assessor, it is inappropriate to be overly friendly with a student you supervise or assess. Social networking with someone while you are also supporting them in a professional capacity is a potential risk to your registration. Reflecting on this, it would be beneficial for both parties to inform themselves about policies and guidance on using media within the organisation and from a regulation perspective. *The Code* (NMC, 2018b), in the section *Promote professionalism and trust* (item 20.3), explicitly identifies this and refers the reader to their online guidance (**www.nmc-uk.org/guidance**). Reading through this section, you will note that other items (20.5–20.8) are also relevant to these scenarios. Other aspects of *The Code* (NMC, 2018b) about confidentiality and protecting personal rights are also applicable and it is strongly recommended that in addition you consider Case studies 10.2 and 10.3 from these broader perspectives of professional practice.

### Activity 10.3 Reflection

The script might go as follows:

'Get out, you stupid woman!', he shouted, raising his fist at his sister. I hurriedly ushered her out of the room and then went back to try to calm him down. He had come to the unit after smashing up his home and threatening the police and his family. For the last 3 weeks I had been trying to build up a therapeutic relationship with him to get him to communicate and come out of himself more. I had not intended for him to react like this, though, when I told his sister he was ready to see her. I should have been scared, but I felt calm. He was out of control, but I felt in control of the situation. The preparation I have had has, I think, helped me feel this way. What would I have done if he hit me? Others might say, 'It is your own fault because you did not ask for help'. I would have to rethink my strategy. But for now, things are calming down. I go home feeling great after the glowing report from my practice supervisor. My communication strategies have been rewarded and affirmed by the patient calming down and my practice supervisor praising my handling of the situation. I feel ready to progress towards being a qualified nurse.

## Further reading

**Allcot, H., Braghieri, L., Eichmeyer, S. & Gentzkow, M.** (2020). The welfare effects of social media. *American Economic Review,* 110(3), 629–676. https://pubs.aeaweb.org/doi/pdfplus/10.1257/aer.20190658

This article looks at the possible negative effects of social media and the potential benefits of reducing time spent on Facebook.

**Donaldson, I. & Cooper, K.** (2020). Introducing an online portfolio for practice placement assessments. *Nursing Times,* 116(2), 59–62. www.nursingtimes.net/roles/nurse-educators/introducing-an-online-portfolio-for-practice-placement-assessments-20-01-2020/

This article describes an initiative in applying e-portfolios to enhance the assessment of nursing students' clinical skills.

## Useful websites

**www.creativementalhealth2025.blogspot.com**

A highly creative blog using new media to write and reflect personally and professionally by Steve McG.

**www.learninghub.nhs.uk**

The Learning Hub provides access to eLearning, specialist health and care content which has been developed by the Royal Colleges, universities and other health and care organisations.

**www.onlinepare.net**

Designed in 2013 as a digital practice assessment document.

**www.patientvoices.org.uk**

This website offers useful stories involving patients and nurses in diverse settings and situations. You might find it helpful to access the website **https://www.nurstory.org/stories/** to develop your ideas.

**www.rcn.org.uk**

The RCN website offers advice and guidance on issues relating to nursing. It also has discussion forums where nurses can share practice.

# Chapter 11 Critical reflection

## NMC Future Nurse: Standards of Proficiency for Registered Nurses

This chapter will address the following platforms and proficiencies:

**Platform 1: Being an accountable professional**

1.5 Understand the demands of professional practice and demonstrate how to recognise signs of vulnerability in themselves or their colleagues and the action required to minimise risks to health.

1.17 Take responsibility for continuous self-reflection, seeking and responding to support and feedback to develop their professional knowledge and skills.

**Platform 5: Leading and managing nursing care and working in teams**

5.6 Exhibit leadership potential by demonstrating an ability to guide, support and motivate individuals and interact confidently with other members of the care team.

5.10 Contribute to supervision and team reflection activities to promote improvements in practice and services.

## Chapter aims

After reading this chapter you will be able to:

- critically examine personal contributions and those of others within practical and psychological considerations;
- explore the limits of your understanding;
- assess sources of evidence within any situation;
- identify the coming together of new ideas.

## Case Study 11.1: Meg gives first aid

Meg was in the third year of her adult nursing degree programme. On her way home from placement, she stopped at the supermarket. Suddenly she heard a thump behind her, and she saw a man drop to the floor. Meg placed him in the recovery position and observed that he appeared rigid and was **cyanosed**. Meg recognised this as the **tonic** phase of an **epileptic seizure** and cleared a space around him so that, as the **clonic** phase of jerking started, he would not injure himself. Meg continued to monitor that he started breathing again as the tonic phase gave way to the clonic phase. At this point customers had gathered around, and someone said that he was a first aider and that she should put something between the man's teeth to stop him biting his tongue. Meg was not sure whether this was right and decided not to follow the advice even though the man was insistent. The staff had called an ambulance and, when the paramedics arrived, Meg told them what she had done.

When she got home, she found that she felt quite shaken by what had happened and wondered why she was feeling this way. She realised that this was a reaction to the adrenaline rush she had experienced and, although it had helped to focus her mind on what was important, it had caused her current physiological reaction.

Later that evening, Meg was able to critically reflect on her actions. In hindsight, she could have checked the man for other signs, such as looking at his pupils and checking for any injury, as there could be several reasons why someone might have a seizure. She was satisfied to have maintained the man's airway and that she had immediately placed him in the recovery position. Meg thought of what the alleged first aider had said about placing something between the man's teeth; still unsure, she checked what the nursing literature recommended and found that this action was positively discouraged. Meg was relieved she had not listened and reflected critically on what had led her to this decision. Placing someone in the recovery position is a way to ensure the tongue does not fall back and block the airway so pushing something into the mouth at the same time would likely achieve the opposite effect by forcing the tongue backwards. Meg realised that she had learnt about this earlier in the programme and, although it was not foremost in her mind, it had guided her intuitive response. She realised that, if she had been in the first year of her nursing programme, she might have listened, assuming that the alleged first aider was correct. This led her to reflect on how you could not know the experience, qualifications or knowledge of anyone who stops to help in an emergency and was relieved that she had waited for the ambulance staff. Meg concluded how important it is to work within her own competence and knowledge levels so as not to endanger the patient or herself. She decided that she would do a more thorough initial assessment in future to ensure that she did not miss anything important.

# Introduction

Becoming a professional is about developing criticality to analyse and identify significant priorities and potential solutions. As you progress through your programme you will develop critical skills from first observations to more complex decision-making. In Meg's case she used her initial observations to make decisions about the priorities – the person's airway and safety. Critical reflection enabled her to recognise limitations in her knowledge and ways to remedy these.

This chapter emphasises the importance of critical reflection and its relevance to the developing skill of criticality. It also offers you opportunities to engage in critical reflection through different activities and scenarios. How new ideas come together as the final part of an analytical process are considered at the end.

# Critically examining personal contributions and those of others

In time and with experience, reflective thinking becomes a 'way of being' rather than 'something extra'. One could say that all reflection strives to be critical in that it allows us to examine and question all the factors involved in a situation, which makes the familiar unfamiliar. As discussed in earlier chapters, this means looking at routine situations as if they were new to find out what might be seen differently, and this requires us to maintain focus if we are to achieve the depth of analysis required. Such a questioning approach is also directed at personal actions to investigate motives, assumptions, decision-making and what you were really thinking. The frameworks in Chapter 4 provide structures that can be used to direct a critical approach. Critical reflection, used with critical incident analysis such as reviewing and analysing situations, is important for learning and can help to build case studies from which to learn (Lucas, 2024; Rolfe, 2011). Activities 11.1 and 11.2 help you to begin critical incident analysis and develop your learning by examining your contribution and that of others.

## Activity 11.1 Critical thinking

Critical incident analysis is a form of debrief that looks back at situations to consider what needs to be learnt. For this activity, please review what you have done, or been involved with, in the last few weeks and choose an incident to review. Write a detailed account of the event, including your own and others' actions. Now consider the following questions:

- Why is this situation significant for you?
- How did it affect you?

*(Continued)*

(Continued)

- How did you feel about it?
- What was satisfying about the situation?
- What was concerning about the situation?
- What might you have done differently?
- Was there any additional knowledge that you needed?
- Where might you go to find it?
- What have you learnt?
- How will you take this learning forward?

*There are outline answers to this activity at the end of the chapter.*

### Activity 11.2 Critical thinking

After reviewing your incident, you might like to go further by considering who was responsible and who was accountable in the situation, and any implications in terms of significance, concerns and potential consequences. How does this inform your thinking about being a nurse?

*As this is based on your own experiences, there is no outline answer at the end of the chapter.*

Examining situations in this systematic way may be time consuming, but it ensures that situations are studied for what can be learnt and what can be taken forward as situational and experiential evidence. Connecting this with other forms of knowledge adds to your evidence base. It can be helpful to write a pen portrait of the situation. Writing a pen portrait enables you to bring elements together that are relevant to the situation and the individuals involved, thus providing a complete picture and building on the storytelling we discussed in Chapter 10. A pen portrait should address the following:

- the history and context of the situation;
- your own and others' interpretations and analysis of what was happening;
- your own use of knowledge;
- your own and others' actions and the consequences of those actions;
- insights arising from reflection;
- link of insights to evidence base.

### Case Study 11.2: Anika's pen portrait example

Anika was working on a care for older people ward when Mavis was admitted after a fall. Mavis had been found by her neighbours on the floor, unable to get up. At first, staff assumed she had broken her ankle due to the pain in her foot, but further investigations revealed cellulitis requiring antibiotics. Mavis also had a diagnosis of diabetes, and her blood count showed severe iron-deficiency anaemia. During handover, she was presented as being uncooperative, having refused both analgesia and attempts at rehabilitation. She spent much of her time lying in bed with her eyes closed, while the bed manager was keen for discharge planning to move forward.

From Anika's perspective, however, Mavis appeared exhausted rather than deliberately uncooperative. Through talking with her, Anika noticed that autonomy was clearly very important to Mavis. While some colleagues believed Mavis was not managing her self-care and could not cope independently, Anika's knowledge of psychology suggested that Mavis's resistance stemmed from feeling her autonomy was under threat. Anika felt that adopting a more person-centred approach might yield better results.

When Anika asked Mavis what she wanted, how she wished to achieve it and whether she wanted support from staff, Mavis became more responsive and alert. In contrast, Anika observed that Mavis was less cooperative with colleagues who did not take this approach. Some colleagues dismissed Anika's efforts as a waste of time, but she recognised that Mavis was reacting differently depending on how she was engaged.

Reflecting on the situation, Anika considered that Mavis's resistance was likely due to the sudden loss of autonomy and the lack of consultation in her care. Anika empathised, acknowledging that if she were in Mavis's position, she too might feel frustrated at not being included in decision-making. She concluded that consultation and partnership working were crucial in such cases. While dignity and respect are embedded in professional codes, Anika recognised that subjective judgements about patients still influenced practice. She thought it might be valuable to arrange a lunchtime discussion with colleagues about care, compassion and the principles of the 6 Cs to encourage more reflective and person-centred care.

Healthcare needs to be organised around individuals, not processes, as appears to be happening here. Applying the principles of person-centred care empowers individuals to make choices for themselves and be partners in their care, thereby preparing them to continue in their own environments. In the example above, dignity and respect are mentioned as being part of *The Code* (NMC, 2018b). It is important, however, not to simply name these without exploring them in more detail. Please take time to explore *The NMC Code* and identify which elements would be relevant to Mavis's situation.

Critical incident analysis may be applied to positive and negative situations. Consider the following case study to see how this might be done.

## Case Study 11.3: Elimu's compliment

Elimu was in the final year of his mental nurse apprentice programme and working on an inpatient unit. This was an extended placement, enabling Elimu to get to know the patients and staff and feel a part of the team. He was putting the management principles he was learning into practice when, during a particularly busy shift, one of the patients had a cardiac arrest. Elimu was close by and called for help and then calmly initiated the resuscitation protocol. At the end of the shift his practice supervisor complimented Elimu on his swift actions, calm manner and correct responses.

Elimu thought about this critically on his way home, deconstructing the chain of events and reviewing his actions. He considered whether there were any warning signs he might have missed indicating that the patient was about to arrest, but the observations he had recorded earlier had not changed. Elimu felt that he had responded as quickly as possible and his response was linked to good visual observation of the patients. He had called for help so that the resuscitation team could be alerted and other staff would join him, and this had resulted in someone bringing the necessary equipment. In the meantime, Elimu had started cardio-pulmonary resuscitation because he had learnt how to do this in class. He analysed how different this felt from practising on the simulation mannequin. He needed to concentrate on the amount of force he used to maintain consistency and it was much more tiring than he had anticipated, confirming another reason to seek help.

As part of his management module Elimu had discussed different types of leadership and delegation in a variety of situations, and this knowledge helped him to respond calmly and effectively. However, he recognised that his knowledge of the different drugs that the team used when they arrived was limited. He decided that learning these was something he would take forward from the situation. However, his practice supervisor's compliment had affirmed his actions, and he recognised that these had been appropriate.

The case study identifies the importance of the team in responding to situations and for peer feedback. Interpersonal relationships are important for team building and peer support and can be used for critically examining personal contributions and those of others. Everyone, including the student nurse, relies on peers when entering new clinical environments (Petty, 2014; Williamson et al., 2020). Peer support includes constructive feedback to develop practice, which can be difficult, because it is easy to become critical rather than being critically constructive. Additionally, Lucas (2024) highlights that positive changes regarding emotional well-being for staff of all grades occur when Schwartz Rounds are implemented. By using a structured forum for reflecting together in a 'safe space' and specifically reflecting on social, ethical, and emotional challenges when caring for people (this is also applicable to chapter 8).

Consider Scenario 11.1 and reflect critically on integrating new staff/student into a team.

### Scenario 11.1: Integrating a new member of staff

Recently a new member of staff has joined the team, and she requires constant support, making it difficult for you to get on with your job. You have allocated time to catch up, but she constantly interrupts you for guidance, instead of problem-solving for herself. She is also given exceptional leeway as to flexible working time to accommodate her childcare, which is putting extra pressure on the rest of the team because you must manage after she has left early.

### Activity 11.3 Critical reflection

After critically reflecting on this scenario:

- What do you think are the main reflective points from the perspectives of both the experienced practitioner and the new member of staff?
- What potential learning points have you identified and how might these be applied in practice?

*There are outline answers to these questions at the end of the chapter.*

Trust needs to be developed to facilitate learning critically. Building trust involves three arenas comprising risk, example and consistency (Archer-Kuhn & MacKinnon 2020; Moore, 2023). Reflection and open dialogue are helpful to support trust in sensitive circumstances because students can find integrating into an unknown environment intimidating, whether this is a programme, a new module or a new placement area in practice (Rawson, 2021).

The ability to critically examine personal contributions in relationships with others opens different points of view that are more empathetic and, therefore, supportive of collegial relationships. This leads to a positive atmosphere where it is possible to offer constructive criticism that does not offend people, but from which they learn the limits of their understanding. Mutual understanding and respect allow trust to develop and form the foundation of healthy team relationships.

## Exploring the limits of understanding

Critically reflecting on the limits of our understanding is important for both the novice and experienced practitioner and is enshrined within *The Code* (NMC, 2018b). Even if you were previously competent in a skill or knowledgeable in a particular area, you could become unskilled over time or things could change, meaning that your knowledge and understanding is not current. Healthcare is constantly evolving so things change and new learning is required to maintain your skill set and ensure that you stay abreast of new developments. A critical, reflective stance towards your practice will enable you to identify deficits in your knowledge and skill base and recognise the limits of your understanding. In Chapter 9, we saw that writing reflections facilitates your analysis of experiences, stimulates new ideas and increases awareness of new learning which could, otherwise, remain invisible (Delves-Yates, 2025). Doing this involves critically reviewing daily experience and analysing it, raising awareness of how you are learning and what new knowledge you are developing. Price (2024) suggests that critical thinking requires we continually examine our thinking processes, looking for gaps and identifying supporting evidence and potential consequences of our decisions for others and ourselves.

Price (2024) further defines critical thinking as "A process where different information is gathered, sifted, synthesised and evaluated in order to understand a subject or issue. Critical thinking engages our intellect (the ability to discriminate, challenge and argue), but it might engage our emotions too. To think critically, we need to take account of values, beliefs, and attitudes that shape our perceptions. Critical thinking, then, is that which enables the nurse to function as a knowledgeable practitioner – someone who selects, combines, judges and uses information in order to proceed in a professional manner".

### Case Study 11.4: Rob's dyslexia

Rob was in the first year of his nursing degree programme. It had not been easy for him to learn at school and now the programme was becoming difficult because he had to complete several written assignments.

He reflected critically on the problems he was having with his learning and realised that he could not retain information as well as others could, and this applied to the graduate skills that were expected of him. Rob considered himself good at creative problem-solving and working with people, but he was concerned that he would not be able to function at the same level as other practitioners. Rob realised that, to move forward, he had to overcome his fear and explore the available options.

On reflection, Rob realised that the way he saw things differently was positive because he could see alternative solutions that others could not. He realised that he needed structure to understand new concepts, which was why he found self-directed study challenging. Rob became aware that he made notes to reinforce particular points; handouts were not helpful as he focused on what was being said.

Rob spoke to the study support department at his university and asked his tutors whether he could audio-record their teaching. This meant that he could write down what was important when listening in class and, again, when listening to the recording. In this way he was able to access information more effectively, he had a better idea of what to include in his assignments and it offered him a chance to be reflective.

An example could be thinking about why we react in a particular way in certain situations. To do this, we could analyse our thought processes using a decision-making model in which we question our assumptions. Then we could analyse our thinking using SWOT; by determining strengths, weaknesses, opportunities, and threats, we imagine the possible consequences of thinking in this way.

Undertaking Activity 11.4 can help you to identify limits to your understanding and ways to address these.

## Activity 11.4 Reflection

Please think about a recent situation where you were not sure what to do. Critically reflect on the situation by considering the following questions. Try to structure your reflection using one of the reflective models discussed in Chapter 4.

- What alerted you to the uncertainty?
- What did you know?
- What did you not know?
- What were the consequences?
- What might have been the consequences if you had known?
- What can you do about this?
- What learning do you take from this situation?

*As this activity is based on your own experiences, there is no outline answer at the end of the chapter.*

In this Case Study, Fajid's engagement with Kate could be inhibited by not understanding the context of her role in her family (based on his own life story, as discussed in Chapter 3). This is an important area to explore to be able to reflectively find strategies that work for you.

You may have identified that there are specific areas that you need to learn more about, or that there are some skills that you need to develop or refresh. This is part of being a reflective practitioner and remains core to your professional practice. Now reconsider Activity 11.4 and explore how limited knowledge could, potentially, have posed a safety issue.

## Case Study 11.5: Fajid's understanding of young carers

Fajid was in the first year of his apprentice child nursing programme and on his third placement with the school nurses. His practice supervisor, Simone, involved

*(Continued)*

(Continued)

Fajid in **health promotion** activities, working with schools on healthy eating strategies, and he was involved in vaccination sessions.

Part of the school nurse's role was to support pupils who had behavioural problems and follow up on absenteeism and Simone was currently working with Kate, a young carer for her mum. Simone and Fajid visited Kate at home to assess the situation and find ways to empower her. When he and Simone left the visit, he discussed his concern that a 14-year-old was left caring for her mother as he was accustomed to this being an extended family's responsibility.

In Case Study 11.5, Simone would have helped Fajid's learning by asking him to reflect critically on his approach to Kate's case, the potential consequences of his actions and the breadth of the nurse's professional role. In doing this, we would explore our ability to identify the sources of evidence we use and rectify deficits to maintain safe practice. We now critically assess the sources of evidence in a given situation.

### Activity 11.5 Reflection

- What are the limits to Fajid's understanding in this scenario?
- What might be the consequences for Kate, her mum, and Fajid?

*There is an outline answer to this question at the end of the chapter.*

## Assessing sources of evidence within the situation

An important part of developing our practice at any stage – be that as novice or experienced practitioner – is to reflect critically on the evidence base of our actions to provide good-quality patient care and identify personal learning needs. This means examining which sources of evidence are used when making decisions. Activity 11.6 helps you consider the sources of evidence used in a situation.

### Activity 11.6 Critical thinking

Think of a situation from your experience in practice. Examine the sources of evidence supporting your interpretations and your decision-making, using the following questions:

- How did you assess the situation?
- What was your assessment based on?

- How did you know what to base it on?
- Was your interpretation correct?
- What confirmed that it was correct?
- If it was not correct, what evidence did you have that it was not correct?
- What did you base your subsequent decision on?
- How did you know it was the right decision?

*As this activity is based on your personal experiences, there is an outline answer to only part of this activity at the end of the chapter.*

A useful way of evaluating results from Activity 11.6 is to use a practice development tool called Claims, Concerns and Issues (McCormack et al., 2013; Manley et al., 2014; Olasoji et al., 2021). Claims are favourable assertions about things, Concerns are unfavourable assertions and Issues are questions you might reasonably ask about implementation. Use these terms as headings for three columns and list all your assertions and questions under the appropriate heading. Finally, think about using active questions that will help you to turn issues into positive results. They are a useful guide to ongoing critical reflection.

Confidence to communicate the evidence base for your actions is often subject to the culture in the workplace or the classroom. Lack of managerial or tutor support in situations can reduce cooperation and promote organisational friction. It is important to critically analyse factors such as leadership and your responses to it to identify facilitative and hindering factors that might also affect situations and decision-making.

## Case Study 11.6: Arunda's experience of managing pressure

Arunda was a student in the second year of her adult nursing degree programme, working in an endoscopy suite. The unit was short staffed and had many complex patients to care for. Although Arunda was supposed to be supernumerary, she had to work as a regular member of staff to help them with complex patients. One patient, causing her concern, was an alcoholic who underwent an **oesophageal gastroduodenoscopy (OGD)** procedure that showed that he had oesophageal varices, enlarged veins at the base of his oesophagus. Arunda, responsible for monitoring the patient, alerted the team that his vital signs were changing, and she thought that he had started to bleed. Just before Arunda left, the manager praised her for doing a good job. The following week, in the absence of the manager, Arunda asked her practice supervisor (who had not been present at the emergency) if she could take back some of the time she had used to help with the emergency. Her request was refused, with the practice supervisor saying that Arunda still had a lot to learn in her last week. Arunda met with her university link tutor who asked her how her placement had been. Arunda said it had been tough, but she had learnt a lot.

### Activity 11.7 Reflection

- What sources of evidence might Arunda use to evaluate her learning?
- What sources of evidence was the manager using to evaluate Arunda's learning?
- What sources of evidence was the practice supervisor using to evaluate Arunda's learning?

*There are outline answers to these questions at the end of the chapter.*

When interpretations are not checked for their validity, it is possible for our fears and anxieties to become projected on to another person or situation, and for us to interact with that person or situation as if they meant us harm. Reading the points of guidance suggested at the end of this chapter about Case Studies 11.4 and 11.6, you will notice that the situation can be interpreted in different ways depending on your role, responsibility and experience. Here, critical reflection helps us make sense of the evidence supporting the validity of our interpretations and how ideas fit together.

## Identifying when new ideas come together

Critical reflection offers us psychological space to connect with our ideas and those of others, as well as the mental focus to do so. Our ideas and knowledge may be broad but, to develop, we also need to be open to consider challenging ideas; this means drawing together ideas of process, relationships, caring and ethical behaviour to inform the practice of nursing. Nursing knowledge is interconnected, emerging as a discipline while, as practitioners, we construct our ideas and contribute to this body of nursing knowledge. This role of authorship promotes reflexive dialogue with the ideas obtained from external sources as we progress through our nursing career. This process allows us to develop agency because it also focuses on personal development and practice innovation.

It could be said that lack of feedback reduces the possibility of developing ideas. Therefore, discussing reflections critically with someone is an important part of bringing new ideas together. During your nursing programme, you need the support of peers, practice supervisors, lecturers and clinical colleagues to allow you to develop new ideas of how to act and think as a professional. Even, as experienced practitioners, we need the support of colleagues to challenge and discuss our practice in positive ways because this will stimulate creativity, criticality and imagination. Through this interaction we become proactive in looking for ideas and answers, rather than simply accepting them and maintaining a status quo. These important steps build curiosity, imagination and learning that are life-long and critical.

To illustrate this, Figure 11.1 shows how ideas from the different ways of reflecting that have been discussed throughout this book are brought together. The outer world encompasses learning generated by political systems, organisational structures and scientific enquiry, and is represented by codified knowledge. This learning can be associated with the guidance that is offered, to be internally considered. For example, your practice supervisors and lecturers might identify what you need to learn, give you information and direct you to complete learning tasks. If you are an experienced practitioner, you may be engaging with continuing professional development (CPD) courses or mandatory training, both of which may be prescribed by the employer or registering body. However, only you can make sense of what things mean to you and what you are taking forward through your 'inner-world consideration'.

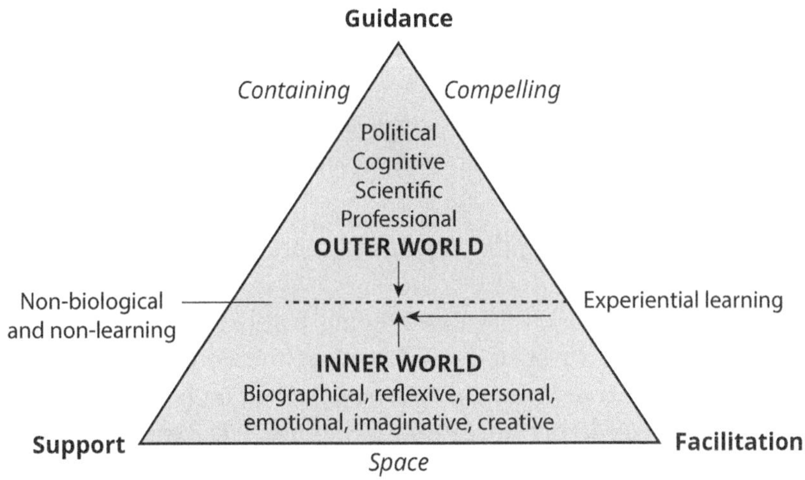


*Figure 11.1* Interrelationships between inner and outer worlds of learning and containing and compelling space (from Howatson-Jones, 2010)

Political, cognitive, scientific and professional ideas are usually consistent with outer-world experiences that intrude on the personal world, where they are met by inner-world sense making. The interface between your outer- and inner-world experience is fluid in that it allows experiences and learning to interact. The inner world encompasses critical learning that helps to internalise experiences and may also be influential in shaping new ones; for example, in the level of self-confidence a person has or their self-esteem. This inner world includes biographical, personal and emotional dimensions, and reflexive, imaginative and creative responses to these dimensions. It is also where your values are embedded. These might relate to the continuous internal dialogue that you have with yourself in response to what is happening externally – namely, your emotional life, which influences your reactions, and biographical memories, which are a part of your sense making, as discussed in Chapter 3.

Experiential learning is located at the interface between inner and outer worlds; in other words, your internal world can influence the outer-world experiences in which you find yourself and vice versa. For example, consider that you are a spontaneous, creative person (inner world); situations where others constantly tell you what you must do and learn can feel constricting and oppressive (outer world). You want to learn to be a professional nurse, so some compromise needs to be reached at the experiential interface between these two worlds. This is where facilitation and support are crucial.

The biographical, personal and emotional dimensions, and reflexive, imaginative and creative responses to these dimensions are influenced by the quality of facilitation and support. These qualities may be included, or excluded, from learning opportunities in environments that are prescriptive. In other words, learning opportunities should link guidance, facilitation and support to help contain anxiety and make learning manageable. Where these are lacking, the interface between inner and outer worlds becomes less fluid, with little chance of critical reflection. The result is non-biographical learning, where nothing is perceived as new, but instead information is just processed with non-awareness and a lack of openness; experiences may be gathered, but nothing is learnt from them. Consider Case Study 11.6 to make sense of these processes.

## Case Study 11.7: Cassie's difficulty with saying no

Cassie had been a care worker in a care home before undertaking her nursing programme. She has always been a good worker and completes tasks to a high standard. In her role as care worker, the manager relied on her and had frequently asked her to help when others would not. Cassie had felt flattered and complied, even though the extra workload caused stress and strained family life.

Cassie had undertaken her nursing programme with the support of her family and throughout the programme, she had tried to maintain her family role and study hard. At one stage she thought of leaving because of the strain she was experiencing. Fortunately, she met with her personal tutor who encouraged Cassie to reflect on what she was doing. This helped her realise that she was taking a passive role, rather than exerting agency in her life. She did not want to be thought of badly by her family or colleagues.

Now, as a newly registered nurse, Cassie felt she needed help to overcome the challenges of having to solve unfamiliar issues and decided to access the clinical supervision offered by her employer. At the first session her clinical supervisor, Annie, asked Cassie to reflect on her journey from being a care worker to becoming a registered nurse. Together they critically examined Cassie's approach to work and noted her tendency to overwork and her inability to say no. Following through the consequences of her choices, Cassie realised that she was not learning from her experiences but was trying to conform to others' views. With Annie's guidance Cassie felt confident enough to acknowledge that she was not a bad person, or nurse, if she refused. In fact, this might sometimes be the responsible thing to do. Cassie continued to reflect long after leaving the session and, as a result, was more considered in approaching problems and caring for herself.

Although reflection may be able to address some of the emotional residues of your work, the critical element is vital to avoid becoming ensnared in narcissistic contemplation that does not move you, or your learning, forward. Honestly exploring the line between inner- and outer-world experience is where awareness of new ideas forms and where you can become aware of what you are learning and how to exert some agency within it. Reflecting on the examples given in this chapter and revisiting *The Code* (NMC, 2018b), it is interesting to discover that explicit reflection on ensuring quality and maintaining boundaries is woven through the different sections of *The NMC Code*. You might want to read the section *Practise effectively* (items 6.2, 8.4, 8.7, 9.1–9.4, 11.1–11.3 and 13.3), the section *Preserve safety* (item 15.1) and the section *Promote professionalism and trust* (items 20.6 and 20.9) to reflect on how *The Code* (NMC, 2018b) could relate to this scenario.

## Chapter summary

Critical reflection is part of being a responsible and accountable practitioner by examining and analysing your practice and learning. As has been noted in this chapter, it requires discipline and systematic thought to critically explore what you are doing, and the evidence base for your interpretations and decisions. These aspects can be missed from simple reflection on practice, which often concentrates on emotional elements. The activities in this chapter offer you an opportunity to complete the cycle of connecting feelings, evidence, decisions and actions through critical reflection that takes an analytical view of your practice and development.

# Brief outline answers

In this section, answers to the chapter's activities will be outlined and explained.

## Activity 11.1 Critical thinking

The incident you describe could have been a mistake or something that went particularly well, but you found it important in developing your practice. For example, a mistake could have created feelings of extreme anxiety, whereas a compliment could have increased your confidence. What you could do differently would probably relate to improving your knowledge, finding out the facts of the case, seeking help and considering how you use communication. Additional knowledge you might have needed could relate to policies and procedures. The learning that you might take forward will potentially relate to communication and decision-making, as well as knowing more about yourself and how you respond to situations. It is important to note that, if the situation were distressing, you might need to reflect on your emotional response first to have emotional closure before you can apply critical reflection to understand aspects of learning in relation to knowledge or skills.

## Activity 11.3 Critical reflection

Perspective of the experienced staff member

As the experienced member of staff, I could ensure that the new colleague has an induction to the department. I could negotiate expectations clearly, identify sources of information and take time to discuss her experience and knowledge. I could arrange points of contact throughout the day to evaluate, which would allow me to remain informed but give the new person the space to make the necessary decisions. This would reduce situations where she need advice because this might undermine her confidence. I should give constructive feedback to boost her confidence. Maybe I am less of a team player than I think and could use emotional intelligence by trying to understand the other person's perspective, rather than focusing on how annoying it is to be disturbed. I am used to working autonomously and therefore find it difficult to adjust. I realise that I expect high personal standards and competence from others, but it is unfair to expect this from a colleague who has recently joined the team. I always thought my management style was democratic, but my standards and expectations may be a controlling influence and could limit someone else's development. Outlining organisational and personal needs may help to clarify concerns and I must be aware that feelings of injustice could cloud the relationship with my new colleague, because she has been able to organise flexible working hours.

Perspective of the new staff member

As a new member of staff, I am anxious about getting things right. I must arrange shifts that are mutually manageable. I am trying to develop my skills through experiencing as much as I can with the support of others, making sure I am doing things correctly. But I am new to this speciality; I feel they think I am a nuisance and that my knowledge is inadequate. I see that the clinical area is busy, and I am embarrassed to ask so many questions but, rather than making a mistake, I want to make sure of what I'm doing. To be effective I need to consider my colleagues' needs as well as my own. Discussing expectations and feedback arrangements might help us to find mutually acceptable solutions to my childcare commitments as well as work requirements.

## Activity 11.5 Reflection

Besides possible cultural differences that may have influenced Fajid, he may assume that healthcare and social care are the same thing. He may not understand that there are costs attached to social care. These are financial as well as personal. Social care needs to be paid for. Some people are also reluctant to have strangers caring for them, especially when it involves personal care. It is natural for Kate to want to help her mother. However, taking on too much is likely to impact on her socially and educationally. Equally, if Fajid is not knowledgeable about why children become carers and about available resources, he cannot help Kate's mother to make different choices because she is the adult in this situation. Fajid may want to consider what the nurse's role is in relation to safeguarding children; one might assume that Kate wants to help her mother, but she may feel that she doesn't have a choice. It would be helpful for Fajid to reflect on these issues with his practice supervisor to fully understand the breadth and depth of healthcare and social care professionals' roles.

## Activity 11.6 Critical thinking

The sources of evidence that you may have used are likely to have included the following:

- objective and subjective data to base your assessment on, such as what you found out through communication, what you observed, what you felt, practice policies and theoretical ideas;
- communication and observation are likely to have confirmed whether your interpretation was correct or identified deficits;
- you may have based your decision-making on a protocol, or an assessment of the alternatives and possible consequences, or on intuition or what you had read;
- how you knew it was the right decision would have been through the feedback of others and what you observed the consequences to be.

## Activity 11.7 Reflection

Arunda might use the evidence of recognising the significance of vital sign changes to demonstrate her knowledge of physiology. She could also consider the manager's praise as showing she works well under pressure. The manager used Arunda's ability to stay calm under pressure and report changes accurately as evidence that she had embedded knowledge. However, this is only in a narrow field and would not necessarily evaluate all the learning that was required of her in this placement. The practice supervisor is likely to take a broader view and may be using the practice learning assessment criteria to evaluate her learning. She may interpret Arunda's request to go home early as evidence that she does not want to learn. Arunda might feel disadvantaged by her practice supervisor refusing her request, but this is important to learn what it is to be a professional. Although not always convenient, there are times when organisational demands are considered above individual wishes. It is understandable that Arunda would have liked to have time off, she could have requested time off. Planning ahead is part of professional practice; once the duty roster has been completed, any absences result in a staff resource gap. As the department is busy, Arunda should have considered these issues before requesting unscheduled time off. This might be interpreted by the practice supervisor as evidence that Arunda is unable to plan adequately, and that she has insufficient insight and overview of staffing management, which could be expected of a second-year student nurse.

## Further reading

**Cottrell, S.** (2023). *Critical thinking skills: Developing effective analysis and argument* (4th ed.). Palgrave Macmillan.

This book can help you to develop the analysis techniques that are a necessary part of critical reflection.

**Ellis, P.** (2025). *Leadership, management and team working in nursing* (5th ed.). Sage/Learning Matters.

This book promotes critical reflection of the importance of teamwork and one's role in contributing to overall care.

**Tappen, R.M., Weiss, S.A. & Whitehead, D.K.** (2010). *Essentials of nursing leadership and management* (5th ed.). FA Davis.

This book can help you to use critical thought in developing in your role, and in developing leadership and management skills.

## Useful websites

**https://nshcs.hee.nhs.uk/wp-content/uploads/2020/08/Guidance-on-critical-reflection-.pdf**

This critical reflection is written by Gillian O'Dell and her experience of dyslexia as a professional nurse.

**https://www.royalmarsdenschool.ac.uk/critical-reflection**

Carole Forde -Johnson says "Student nurses sometimes struggle writing reflective essays and it can take time to develop your academic writing skills. This video provides some simple tips to help you structure your reflective essays and improve your academic writing."

**https://www.youtube.com/watch?v=NTI1nktNmgU**

Nurse Bellinda on how to write critically:

**https://www.youtube.com/watch?v=nQXxk4wFkF8**

# Glossary

**agency** how a person makes use of their life resources to develop strategies for change.

**analgesia** medication that eases pain.

**aortic stent insertion** a tube that is inserted into the aorta to keep the vessel patent and protect the wall of the vessel.

**autobiographical reflection** individuals consider events and experiences throughout life and analyse them to allow self-discovery.

**becoming** a process of change that alters a sense of personal identity.

**biographical** data or written work with focus on an individual's life.

**bullying** attempts to harm, intimidate or coerce someone who is vulnerable.

**catalytic** prompting deep exploration and analysis.

**cathartic** prompting the release of emotion.

**clonic** descriptive of the jerky movements resulting from muscular spasms.

**colonoscopy** an investigative procedure involving passing a flexible tube with a camera through the large bowel to visualise the lining and structure.

**colostomy** where an artificial opening is made and the bowel is brought to the surface to enable the excretion of faeces.

**compelling space** a space that invites a desire to learn in more meaningful ways.

**culture** the meanings and understandings held by a group of people that influence the way they think and act.

**cyanosed** having a lack of oxygen in the tissues, evidenced by a bluish tinge to the lips and fingernails.

**deficit-model** in which individuals are seen as passive recipients of healthcare services, rather than participants in their own health and well-being choices.

**ectopic pregnancy** a fertilised egg that has lodged in the fallopian tube and is at risk of rupturing the tube as it grows.

**empowerment** taking personal control.

**endoscopy** a procedure that visualises the inside of body cavities and tracts using camera technology with a light source and a steerable flexible tube.

**epileptic seizure** a seizure that can manifest itself in a variety of ways and is caused by electrical disruption in the brain.

**e-portfolio** an electronic portfolio that enables a number of different-style documents to be produced, stored and shared.

**espoused theory** evidence-based reasons we give for our nursing actions: nurses have values and beliefs that guide care.

**haemorrhoidectomy** removal of haemorrhoids, which are swollen blood vessels usually located in the anal area.

**health promotion** encouraging people to examine and change their lifestyles to ones that are healthy.

**horizontal violence** 'hostile, aggressive, and harmful behaviour by a nurse or group of nurses towards a co-worker or group of nurses via attitudes, actions, words, and/or other behaviours' (Thobaben, 2007, p. 83).

**intuition/intuitive knowledge** experience-based knowledge.

**learning contract** a plan of learning objectives agreed between the student and the supervisor.

**learning style** a preference for particular ways of learning.

**life world** the history, culture, situations and relationships of an individual.

**lived experience** personal knowledge and experience from directly undergoing a situation, event or way of life.

**losing face** feeling a loss of respect.

**metastases** spread of cells and disease (usually cancer) to another part of the body.

**myomectomy** surgical removal of uterine fibroids.

**oesophageal gastroduodenoscopy (OGD)** a procedure in which a flexible tube with a camera is passed through the oesophagus, stomach and duodenum to visualise the internal lining and structure.

**oncology** cancer care.

**phlebitis** inflammation of a vein.

**prostatectomy** surgical removal of all or part of the prostate gland.

**reflection** considering and reviewing thinking, actions and circumstances to develop new ideas.

**reflection on action** retrospectively analysing a past experience to understand what, why and how it occurred to improve for future practice.

**reflective cycle** a cyclical structuring, review and analysis of thinking, actions and circumstances to develop new ideas, leading to personal and professional growth.

**reflective framework** framing structuring of consideration and review of thinking, actions and circumstances with questions.

**reflective practice** considering and reviewing the interplay between theory and practice and new ideas.

**reflexivity** the conscious engagement on the part of the practitioner to being open to examining their own assumptions and influences on situations, and how the cultures and contexts in which they are embedded might be influencing them.

**robotic-assisted procedure** a surgeon uses a console, with magnified 3D images and robotic instruments; this method is minimally invasive.

**safeguarding reviews** multi-agency review processes to discover what those involved could have done differently that could have prevented harm or a death from taking place.

**self-concept** a perception of who one is and of personal capability.

**self-relience** depending on oneself instead of relying on others.

**socialisation** socialisation is a process of developing meaning through interaction and adaptation.

**Schwartz round** a safe structured forum for clinical and non-clinical healthcare to discuss the emotional and social aspects of their work.

**specific learning differences (SpLD)** an overarching term for several associated learning differences. They affect the way information is learnt and processed, often affecting literacy, memory, coordination and the manipulation of letters and numbers.

**tacit knowledge** knowledge that is so deeply embedded that people often forget they have it. It is known to people within a group and does not need explanation within the context of that group but may be unknown to outsiders.

**theory in use** is actual behaviour in nursing situations, which are not necessarily in accordance with the more formal evidence-based practice **espoused theory**

**tonic** descriptive of muscle rigidity.

**transitional space** where an individual can consider and try out other ways of being.

**trust** management unit of NHS healthcare, which may encompass several providers and settings.

**uterine embolisation** deliberate occlusion of the uterine arteries to terminate blood flow.

**venipuncture** taking a blood sample from a vein.

**virtual meetings** meetings which allow communication over the internet using voice or video contact so that you can see each other face to face.

# References

Alheit, P. (2018). Biographical learning – within the lifelong learning discourse. In K. Illeris (Ed.), *Contemporary theories of learning: Learning theorists... in their own words* (pp. 153–165). Routledge.

Alt, D., Raichel, N., & Naamati-Schneider, L. (2022). Higher education students' reflective journal writing and lifelong learning skills: Insights from an exploratory sequential study. *Frontiers in Psychology, 12*, 707168. https://doi.org/10.3389/fpsyg.2021.707168

Andrew, N., McGuinness, C., Reid, G., & Corcoran, T. (2009). Greater than the sum of its parts: Transition into the first year of undergraduate nursing. *Nurse Education in Practice, 9*(1), 13–21. https://doi.org/10.1016/j.nepr.2008.05.001

Andrew, N., Tolson, D., & Ferguson, D. (2008). Building on Wenger: Communities of practice in nursing. *Nurse Education Today, 28*(3), 246–252. https://doi.org/10.1016/j.nedt.2007.05.002

Archer-Kuhn, B., & MacKinnon, S. (2020). Inquiry-based learning in higher education: A pedagogy of trust. *Journal of Education and Training Studies, 8*(9), 1–14. https://doi.org/10.11114/jets.v8i9.4929

Argyris, C., & Schön, D. (1978). *Organisational learning: A theory of action perspective.* Addison-Wesley.

Artioli, G., Deiana, L., De Vincenzo, F., Raucci, M., Amaducci, G., Bassi, M. C., Di Leo, S., Hayter, M., & Ghirotto, L. (2021). Health professionals and students' experiences of reflective writing in learning: A qualitative meta-synthesis. *BMC Medical Education, 21*(1), 394.

Atkins, S., & Murphy, K. (1995). Reflective practice. *Nursing Standard, 9*(45), 31–37.

Aydogdu, A. L. F., & Disbudak, B. (2025). Interpersonal conflicts in nursing through the lens of senior nursing students: A qualitative study. *Nurse Education Today, 144*, 105741.

Banks, J. A., Au, K. H., Ball, A. F., Bell, P., Gordon, E. W., Gutiérrez, K. D., Brice Heath, S., Lee, C. D., Lee, Y., Mahiri, J., Suad Nasir, N., Valdes, G., & Zhou, M. (2007). *Learning in and out of school in diverse environments: Life-long, life-wide, life-deep.* The LIFE Center.

Barchard, F. (2022). Exploring the role of reflection in nurse education and practice. *Nursing Standard, 37*(6), 45–49.

Barksby, J., Butcher, N., & Whysall, A. (2015). A new model of reflection for clinical practice. *Nursing Times, 111*(34–35), 21–23.

Beck, M. S., & Neil, J. A. (2021). Digital storytelling: A qualitative study exploring the benefits, challenges, and solutions. *CIN: Computers, Informatics, Nursing, 39*(3), 123–128.

Benner, P. (1984). *From novice to expert: Excellence and power in clinical nursing practice.* Addison-Wesley.

Bhabha, H. K. (2012). *The location of culture* (2nd ed.). Routledge.

Bishop, V. (2017). *Clinical supervision in practice* (2nd ed.). Palgrave Macmillan.

Bjerkvik, L. K., & Hilli, Y. (2019). Reflective writing in undergraduate clinical nursing education: A literature review. *Nurse Education in Practice, 35*, 32–41.

Bolton, G., & Delderfield, R. (2018). *Reflective practice: Writing and professional development* (5th ed.). Sage.

Boud, D., Keogh, R., & Walker, D. (Eds.) (1985). *Reflection: Turning experience into learning.* Kogan Page.

Boud, D., & Miller, N. (2002). *Working with experience: Animating learning.* Routledge.

Boyd, C. (2023). *Reflective practice for nurses.* Wiley-Blackwell.

Brechin, A. (2000). Introducing critical practice. In A. Brechin, H. Brown, & A. Eby (Eds.), *Critical practice in health and social care* (pp. 25–47). SAGE.

Brookfield, S. (2005). *The power of critical theory for adult learning and teaching.* Open University Press.

Buckley, A. R. (2025). The moral maze: Navigating the ethical landscape of healthcare. *British Journal of Nursing, 34*(12), 650–656.

Buckley, A. R., Corless, L., Crowle, A., Gallacher, J., & Watkinson, K. (2024a). Narratives: A powerful tool in nurse education and practice. *Nursing Times, 120*(9). https://www.nursingtimes.net/education-and-training/narratives-a-powerful-tool-in-nurse-education-and-practice-05-08-2024/

Buckley, A. R., Corless, L., Crowle, A., Taylor, A., & Warren, E. (2024b). Turning the lens on ourselves: Exploring the practitioner's own narrative. *Nursing Times, 120*(12). https://www.nursingtimes.net/education-and-training/turning-the-lens-on-ourselves-exploring-the-practitioners-own-narrative-11-11-2024/

Bulman, C., & Schutz, S. (Eds.) (2013). *Reflective practice in nursing.* John Wiley & Sons.

Carper, B. (1978). Fundamental patterns of knowing in nursing. *Advances in Nursing Science, 1*(1), 13–23.

Chackal, T., & Mitchell, C. (2025). Violence facing nurses and the threats they pose to autonomy and justice. *Nursing Ethics.* Advance online publication. https://doi.org/10.1177/09697330251317671

Chan, E. A., & Schwind, J. K. (2006). Two teachers reflect on acquiring their nursing identity. *Reflective Practice,* 7(3), 303–314.

Cheraghi, R., Parizad, N., Alinejad, V., Piran, M., & Almasi, L. (2025). The effect of emotional intelligence on nurses' job performance: The mediating role of moral intelligence and occupational stress. *BMC Nursing, 24,* 1–12.

Coleman, D., & Willis, D. S. (2015). Reflective writing: The student nurse's perspective on reflective writing and poetry writing. *Nurse Education Today, 35*(7), 906–911.

Connor, J., Flenady, F., Dwyer, T., & Massey, D. (2025). Acknowledging: A classic grounded theory explaining how nurses employ clinical judgement when complying with early warning system protocols. *International Journal of Nursing Studies, 163*, Article 104567.

Cronin, C., & Hawthorne, C. (2019). Poetry in motion' a place in the classroom: Using poetry to develop writing confidence and reflective skills. *Nurse Education Today, 76*, 73–77.

Davis, N., Clark, A. C., O'Brien, M., Plaice, C., Sumpton, K., & Waugh, S. (2011). *Learning skills for nursing students.* Learning Matters.

de Vries, J., & Timmins, F. (2016). Care erosion in hospitals: Problems in reflective nursing practice and the role of cognitive dissonance. *Nurse Education Today, 38*, 5–8.

Delves-Yates, C. (2025). *Beginner's guide to reflective practice in nursing* (2nd ed.). Sage.

Department of Health. (1997). *The Caldicott Committee report on the review of patient identifiable information.* HMSO.

Department of Health. (2008). *A high quality workforce.* HMSO.

Department of Health. (2009). *The NHS constitution: Securing the NHS today for generations to come.* HMSO.

Department of Health. (2012). *Compassion in practice.* Department of Health.

Department of Health. (2015). *A consultation on updating the NHS constitution.* HMSO.https://www.gov.uk/government/uploads/system/uploads/attachment_data/file/417637/Update_NHS_Constitution.pdf

Department of Health. (2025). *Fit for the future: NHS 10-year health plan for England.* HMSO. https://www.gov.uk/government/publications/10-year-health-plan-for-england-fit-for-the-future/fit-for-the-future-10-year-health-plan-for-england-accessible-version#chapter-8-powering-transformation—innovation-to-drive-healthcare-reform

Department of Health & NHS Commissioning Board. (2012). *Compassion in practice.* Department of Health.

Dewey, J. (1933). *How we think: A restatement of reflective thinking to the educative process.* D. C. Heath.

Dimonte, V., Luciani, M., Conti, A., Malinverni, E., Clari, M., Campagna, S., & Garrino, L. (2021). Nursing students' perspectives of dance movement therapy to learn relational skills: A qualitative description study. *Nurse Education Today, 97.* Article 104707.

Dominice, P. (2000). *Learning from ourselves.* Jossey-Bass.

Driscoll, J. (2007). *Practising clinical supervision: A reflective approach for healthcare professionals* (2nd ed.). Baillière-Tindall.

Edwards, S. (2017). Reflecting differently. New dimensions: Reflection-before-action and reflection-beyond-action. *International Practice Development Journal, 4*(2), 1–14.

Ellis, P. (2022). *Evidence-based practice in nursing* (5th ed.). Sage.

Ellis, P. (2025a). *Understanding ethics for nursing students* (2nd ed.). Sage.

Ellis, P. (2025b). *Leadership, management and team working in nursing* (5th ed.). Sage.

Farrell, G. (2001). From tall poppies to squashed weeds. *Journal of Advanced Nursing, 35*, 26–33.

Faugier, J., & Butterworth, T. (1994). *Clinical supervision: A position paper.* Manchester: University of Manchester.

Field, J. (2006). *Lifelong learning and the new educational order* (2nd ed.). Trentham Books.

Fischer-Rosenthal, W. (2000). Biographical work and biographical structuring in present-day stories. In P. Chamberlayne, J. Bornat, & T. Wengraf (Eds.), *The turn to biographical methods in social science: Comparative issues and examples* (pp. 109–125). Routledge.

Fish, S., Johnson, F., & Pearson, F. (2023). *Safeguarding adults review Whorlton Hall.* https://www.safeguardingdurhamadults.info/media/42270/Safeguarding-Adults-Review-Whorlton-Hall-May-2023/pdf/WhorltonHallReport-May2023.pdf?m=638205410398630000

Fontaine, D. K., Cunningham, T., & May, N. (2024). *Self-care for new and student nurses.* Sigma Theta Tau.

Francis, R. (2013). *Report of the Mid Staffordshire NHS Foundation Trust public inquiry: Executive summary.* HMSO. https://www.midstaffspublicinquiry.com/sites/default/files/report/Executive%20summary.pdf

Francis, R., & Power, R. (2023). Letter to the secretary of state. *Patients' Association.* https://www.patients-association.org.uk/news/declare-a-national-incident

Freshwater, D. (2000). Crosscurrents: Against cultural narration in nursing. *Journal of Advanced Nursing, 32*(2), 481–484.

Freshwater, D., Walsh, E., & Esterhuizen, P. (2007). Models of effective and reflective teaching and learning for best practice. In V. Bishop (Ed.), *Clinical supervision in practice: Some questions, answers and guidelines for professionals in health and social care* (2nd ed.). Palgrave Macmillan.

Froneman, K., du Plessis, E., & van Graan, A. C. (2023). A concept analysis of facilitating presence through guided reflection for transformative learning in nursing education. *Nursing Open, 10*(5), 2920–2933.

Geltmeyer, K., Duprez, V., Blondeel, M., Serraes, B., Eeckloo, K., & Malfait, S. (2025). The effect of different care delivery models in a hospital setting on patient- and nurse-related outcomes: A systematic review with narrative synthesis. *Journal of Advanced Nursing, 81*(1), 140–155. https://doi.org/10.1111/jan.16271

Geoghan Marold, S. M., Strouse, S. M., & Butcher, D. (2025). Professional identity in nursing: A narrative review of the ISPIN definition and domains usage. *Sage Open Nursing, 11.* https://doi.org/10.1177/23779608251335240

Gibbs, G. (1988). *Learning by doing: A guide to teaching and learning methods (RP 391).* FEU.

Gleeson, L., O'Brien, G. L., O'Mahony, D., & Byrne, S. (2023). Interprofessional communication in the hospital setting: A systematic review of the qualitative literature. *Journal of Interprofessional Care, 37*(2), 203–213.

Gobbi, M. (2021). The hidden curriculum': Learning the tacit and embodied nature of nursing practice. In *Work-based learning in clinical settings* (pp. 103–124). CRC Press.

Greenwood, T. J. N. (2011). Professional resource: Digital storytelling in the classroom: New media pathways to literacy, learning, and creativity (2008). *Journal of Media Literacy Education, 3*(2), 134–136.

Habermas, J. (1971). *Knowledge and human interests.* Heinemann.

Hakvoort, L., Dikken, J., Cramer – Kruit, J., Molendijk- van Nieuwenhuyzen, K., van der Schaaf, M., &Schuurmans, M. (2022). Factors that influence continuing professional development over a nursing career: A scoping review. *Nurse Education in Practice, 65.* Article 103481.

Hargreaves, J. (2004). So how do you feel about that? Assessing reflective practice. *Nurse Education Today, 24*(3), 196–201.

Hawkins, P., & Shohet, R. (Eds.) (1989). *Supervision in the helping professions.* Open University Press.

Health and Care Act. (2022). https://www.legislation.gov.uk/ukpga/2012/7/contents/enacted

Hertz, R. (Ed.) (1997). *Reflexivity and voice.* Sage.

Hewitt, O. (2014). A survey of experiences of abuse. *Tizard Learning Disability Review, 19*(3), 122–129.

Hopkins, J. F., Hamilton, B. E., Prematunga, R. K., Ennis, G., Fairest, K., & Houghton, J. (2021). Action learning sets for supporting postgraduate mental health nurses' transition to professional practice: A qualitative study. *International Journal of Mental Health Nursing, 30*(3), 772–782.

Horn, A., & Jackson, A. (2025). *C-bar model reflective practice.* You-tube. https://www.youtube.com/@CBar-model

Horowitz, S. A. (2018). The discovery and loss of a "compelling space": A case study in adapting to a new organizational order. In *Working below the surface* (pp. 151–163). Routledge.

Horsdal, M. (2012). *Telling lives: Exploring dimensions of narratives.* Routledge.

Horton-Deutsch, S., & Sherwood, G. (2024). *Reflective practice: Reimagining ourselves, reimagining nursing* (3rd ed.). Nursing Knowledge International.

Hover, L. A., & Williams, G. B. (2022). New nurses' experience with lateral violence and their decision to remain in nursing. *International Journal for Human Caring, 26*(4), 199.

Howatson-Jones, L. (2010). *Exploring the learning of nurses* (Unpublished PhD thesis, Canterbury Christ Church University/University of Kent).

Howatson-Jones, L. (2023a). Ethical aspects of patient assessment dilemmas. In L. Howatson-Jones, M. Standing, & S. Roberts (Eds.), *Patient assessment and care planning in nursing* (4th ed., pp. 108–120). Sage.

Howatson-Jones, L. (2023b). Making sense of patient information. In L. Howatson-Jones, M. Standing, & S. Roberts (Eds.), *Patient assessment and care planning in nursing* (4th ed., pp. 33–50). Sage.

Howatson-Jones, L., & Thurgate, C. (2014). Biographical learning: A process for recovering the soul in nursing. In L. Formenti, L. West, & M. Horsdal (Eds.), *Embodied narratives: Connecting stories, bodies, cultures and ecologies* (pp. 255–273). University Press of Southern Denmark.

Hunt, C., & West, L. (2007). Salvaging the self in adult learning: Auto/biographical perspectives from teaching and research. In *Paper presented at the conference of the ESREA network on life history and biography, Roskilde University, Denmark.*

Hutchinson, M., Vickers, M., Jackson, D., & Wilkes, L. (2006). Workplace bullying in nursing: Towards a more critical organisational perspective. *Nursing Inquiry, 13*(2), 118–126.

Iedema, R. (2011). Creating safety by strengthening clinicians' capacity for reflexivity. *BMJ Quality and Safety, 20*(Suppl. 1), i83–i86.

Illeris, K. (Ed.) (2009). *Contemporary theories of learning: Learning theorists in their own words.* Routledge.

Jackson, J. D. (2025). Using emotional awareness to facilitate reflection in nursing practice. *Nursing Standard, 40*(6), 68–73.

Jakobsen, L. M., & Sunde Mæhre, K. (2023). Can a structured model of ethical reflection be used to teach ethics to nursing students? An approach to teaching nursing students a tool for systematic ethical reflection. *Nursing Open, 10*(2), 721–729.

Jarvis, P. (2006) Towards a comprehensive theory of human learning. In *Lifelong learning and the learning society* (*Vol. 1*). Routledge.

Jarvis, P. (2007) Globalisation, lifelong learning and the learning society: Sociological perspectives. In *Lifelong learning and the learning society* (*Vol. 2*). Routledge.

Jarvis, P. (2024). *Adult education and lifelong learning: Theory and practice* (5th ed.). Routledge.

Jasper, M. (2003). *Beginning reflective practice.* Nelson Thornes.

Johns, C. (1995). Framing learning through reflection within Carper's fundamental ways of knowing in nursing. *Journal of Advanced Nursing, 22,* 226–234.

Johns, C. (2010). *Guided reflection: A narrative approach to advancing professional practice* (2nd ed.). Wiley-Blackwell.

Johns, C. (2012). How holistic are we? The role of narrative, storytelling and reflection in the development of holistic practice. *European Journal of Cancer Care, 21,* 561–564.

Johns, C. (2013). *Becoming a reflective practitioner* (4th ed.). John Wiley.

Johns, C. (Ed.) (2025). *Becoming a reflective practitioner* (7th ed.). Wiley.

Johns, C., & Freshwater, D. (Eds.) (2005). *Transforming nursing through reflective practice* (2nd ed.). Blackwell.

Jones, R. (2019). *10 tips for using social media to progress your career.* RCN. https://www.rcn.org.uk/magazines/bulletin/2019/january/10-top-tips-for-using-social-media

Jones, S. (2023). Let's start treating clinical supervision like it's an essential. *Nursing Standard, 38*(3), 26–27.

Junious, D. L., & Cain, R. (2025). The impact of emotional intelligence among a multigenerational workforce. *Nursing Administration Quarterly, 49*(2), 123–129.

Kolb, D. (1984). *Experiential learning: Experience as the source of learning and development.* Prentice Hall. https://www.researchgate.net/publication/235701029_Experiential_Learning_Experience_as_the_Source_of_Learning_and_Development/link/00b7d52aa908562f9f000000/download

Kolb, A. Y., & Kolb, D. (2013). *The KOLB learning style inventory, version 4.0: A comprehensive guide to the theory, psychometrics, research on validity and educational applications.* Experience Based Learning Systems. https://learningfromexperience.com/downloads/research-library/the-kolb-learning-style-inventory-4-0.pdf

Kotera, Y., Cockerill, V., Chircop, J., Kaluzeviciute, G., & Dyson, S. (2021). Predicting self-compassion in UK nursing students: Relationships with resilience, engagement, motivation, and mental wellbeing. *Nurse Education in Practice, 51,* Article 102989.

Lachman, V. D. (2016). Moral resilience: Managing moral distress and moral residue. *Medsurg Nursing, 25*(2), 121–124.

Lee, E. J. (2020). Authenticity model of (mass-oriented) computer mediated communication: Conceptual explorations and testable propositions. *Journal of Computer-Mediated Communication, 25*(1), 60–73.

Lee, D., & Suh, E. E. (2025). Development and application of a storytelling-based burn care education program for nursing students. *Nurse Education Today,* Article 106787.

Levi, D., & Askay, D. A. (2025). *Group dynamics for teams.* Sage.

Levy-Malmberg, R., Boman, E., Lehwaldt, D., Fagerström, L., & Lockwood, E. B. (2024). Clinical decision-making processes among graduate nurses, specialist nurses and nurse practitioners: A collaborative international study. *International Nursing Review, 71*(2), 224–231.

Leyden, K., Campbell-Law, L., Nguyen, L., & Piazza, M. D. (2018). Creative reflections: How students find meaning in unexpected clinical experiences. *Journal of Comprehensive Nursing Research and Care, 3,* 131–136.

London, M., Sessa, V. I., & Shelley, L. A. (2023). Developing self-awareness: Learning processes for self-and interpersonal growth. *Annual Review of Organizational Psychology and Organizational Behavior, 10,* 261–288.

Loughran, J. J. (2002). Effective reflective practice: In search of meaning in learning about teaching. *Journal of Teacher Education, 53*(1), 33–43.

Lucas, B. (2024). How to reflect on clinical practice. *Nursing Standard.* Advance online publication. https://doi.org/10.7748/ns.2024.e12365

Mahon, P., & O'Neill, M. (2020). Through the looking glass: The rabbit hole of reflective practice. *British Journal of Nursing, 29*(13), 777–783.

Manley, K., O'Keefe, H., Jackson, C., Pearce, J., & Smith, S. (2014). A shared purpose framework to deliver person-centred, safe and effective care: Organisational transformation using practice development methodology. *International Practice Development Journal, 4*(1), Article 2. http://www.fons.org/Resources/Documents/Journal/Vol4No1/IPDJ_0401_02.pdf

Martlew, C. (2023). The five stages of reflective thinking: What we can still learn from John Dewey. *LinkedIn.* http://www.linkedin.com/pulse/five-stages-reflective-thinking-what-we-can-still-learn-clive-martlew

Matthews-DeNatale, G. (2013). Digital story-making in support of student meaning-making. In *Enhancing instruction with visual media: Utilizing video and lecture capture* (pp. 192–203). IGI Global.

McAndrew, S., & Roberts, D. (2015). Reflection in nurse education: Promoting deeper thinking through the use of painting. *Reflective Practice, 16*(2), 206–217.

McCarthy, B., McCarthy, J., Trace, A., & Grace, P. (2016). Addressing ethical concerns arising in nursing and midwifery students' reflective assignments. *Nursing Ethics, 25*(6), 1–13.

McClunie-Trust, P., Jarden, R., Marriot, P., Winnington, R., Dewar, J., Shannon, K., Jones, S., Jones, V., Turner, R., Cochrane, L., & Macdiarmid, R. (2024). Graduate entry nursing students' development of professional nursing self: A scoping review. *Nurse Education Today, 151,* 104670.

McClunie-Trust, P., Macdiarmid, R., Jones, V., Marriot, P., Winnington, R., Shannon, K., Dewar, J. & Jarden, R. J. (2025). Graduate entry nursing students' development of professional nursing self: A longitudinal case study. *Nurse Education Today, 151,* 106722.

McCormack, B., Manley, K., & Titchen, A. (2013). *Practice development in nursing and healthcare* (2nd ed.). Wiley-Blackwell.

Moon, J. (2000). *Reflection in learning and professional development: Theory and practice.* Kogan Page.

Moore, A. K. (2023). Storytelling: Manifesting integral interconnectedness in holistic nursing education. *Journal of Holistic Nursing, 41*(4), 403–410.

Nåden, D., & Eriksson, K. (2000). The phenomenon of confirmation: An aspect of nursing as an art. *International Journal for Human Caring, 4*(3), 23–28.

Nåden, D., & Eriksson, K. (2002). Encounter: A fundamental category of nursing as an art. *International Journal for Human Caring, 6*(1), 34–40.

National Institute for Health and Care Excellence (NICE). (2021). *Clinical guideline: Autism spectrum disorder in adults: Diagnosis and management.* https://www.nice.org.uk/guidance/cg142

National Society for the Prevention of Cruelty to Children (NSPCC). (2018). *Gillick competency and Fraser guidelines: Balancing children's rights with the responsibility to keep them safe from harm.* NSPCC Knowledge and Information Services. https://learning.nspcc.org.uk/media/1541/gillick-competency-factsheet.pdf

NHS England. (2025). *Learning from lives and deaths – people with a learning disability and autistic people.* https://www.england.nhs.uk/learning-disabilities/improving-health/learning-from-lives-and-deaths/

NHS Resolution. (2025). *About NHS resolution.* https://resolution.nhs.uk/about/

Nieuwerburgh, C. V., & Love, D. (2025). *Your essential guide to effective reflective practice: Improving practice through self-reflection and writing.* Sage.

Nightingale, F. (1969). *Notes on nursing: What it is and what it is not.* Dover.

Nihei, Y., Asakura, K., Sugiyama, S., & Takada, N. (2022). A concept analysis of shame in the field of nursing. *Nursing Forum, 57*(6), 1529–1535.

Noble, C., Ajjawi, R., Billett, S., & Goldszmidt, M. (2025). How to approach qualitative observational research in workplace learning. *The Clinical Teacher, 22*(1), e70005.

Nursing and Midwifery Council (NMC). (2006). *Clinical supervision.* NMC.

Nursing and Midwifery Council. (2017). *Revalidation: How to revalidate with the NMC requirements for renewing your registration.* NMC.

Nursing and Midwifery Council. (2018a). *Future nurse: Standards of proficiency for registered nurses.* NMC.

Nursing and Midwifery Council. (2018b). *The code: Professional standards of practice and behaviour for nurses and midwives.* NMC.

Nursing and Midwifery Council. (2019). *How to revalidate with the NMC: Requirements for renewing your registration.* NMC.

Nursing and Midwifery Council. (2024). *Standards framework for nursing and midwifery education.* https://www.nmc.org.uk/standards-for-education-and-training/standards-framework-for-nursing-and-midwifery-education/

Nursing and Midwifery Council. (2025). *Social media guidance: Our guidance on the use of social media.* https://www.nmc.org.uk/standards/guidance/social-media-guidance/

O'Connor, S., Odewusi, T., Smith, P. M., & Booth, R. G. (2022). Digital professionalism on social media: The opinions of undergraduate nursing students. *Nurse Education Today, 111*, 105322.

Ohler, J. (2008). *Digital storytelling in the classroom: New media pathways to literacy, learning and creativity.* Corwin Press.

Olasoji, M., Plummer, V., & Cross, W. (2021). Strategies for implementing consumer involvement in nursing handover on acute mental health in-patient units. *Issues in Mental Health Nursing, 42*(10), 951–959.

Padykula, B. M. (2017). RN-BS students' reports of their self-care and health-promotion practices in a holistic nursing course. *Journal of Holistic Nursing, 35*(3), 221–246.

Palmer, A., Burns, S., & Bulman, C. (1994). *Reflective practice in nursing: The growth of the professional practitioner.* Blackwell Scientific.

Parse, R. R. (2004). A human becoming teaching–learning model. *Nursing Science Quarterly, 17*(1), 33–35.

Pereira, R. A. M., & Sousa Valente Ribeiro, P. C. P. (2023). Ways and means to comfort people at the end of life: How is the nurse a privileged player in this process? *Palliative Care and Social Practice, 17,* 26323524231182730.

Petty, G. (2014). *Teaching today: A practical guide* (5th ed.). Oxford University Press.

Pierson, W. (1998). Reflection and nursing education. *Journal of Advanced Nursing, 27,* 165–170.

Price, B. (2024). *Critical thinking and writing in nursing* (6th ed.). Learning Matters, Sage Publishing.

Quality Assurance Agency (QAA). (2024). *The UK quality code for higher education.* https://www.qaa.ac.uk/the-quality-code/2024

Rafferty, A. M., & Leary, A. (2023). Nursing notes on a scandal. *Future Healthcare Journal, 10*(1), 3–6.

Rawson, R. (2021). How to integrate into a clinical placement team: Tips on preparing well and staying focused to improve your chances of a positive placement. *Nursing Standard.* https://rcni.com/nursing-standard/students/clinical-placements/how-to-integrate-a-clinical-placement-team-175976

Reed, S. (2015). *Successful professional portfolios for nursing students* (2nd ed.). Learning Matters, Sage Publishing.

Robinson, S., & Doody, O. (2022). *Nursing & healthcare ethics* (6th ed.). Elsevier.

Rogers, C., & Freiberg, H. J. (1994). *Freedom to learn* (3rd ed.). Macmillan College.

Rolfe, G. (Ed.) (2011). *Critical reflection in practice: Generating knowledge for caring* (2nd ed.). Palgrave.

Royal College of Nursing (RCN). (2009). *Legal advice for RCN members using the internet.* https://portal.yhcs.org.uk/documents/70038/70340/Royal+College+of+Nursing+-+Internet+Guidance.pdf/8445a2ca-7873-4e3c-8bb7-450813b9ec45

Royal College of Nursing (RCN). (2019). *RCN social media policy 2019.* RCN.

Royal College of Nursing (2023). *Social media: 5 ways it can benefit you (and 5 ways to protect yourself).* https://www.rcn.org.uk/magazines/Advice/2023/Oct/Social-media-5-ways-it-can-benefit-you-and-5-ways-to-protect-yourself

Ruyak, S., Wright, M., & Levi, A. (2017). Simulation to meet curricular needs in ethics. *Clinical Simulation in Nursing, 13*(3), 121–126.

Schmidt, N. A. (2008). Guided imagery as internally orientated self-care: A nursing case. *Self-Care, Dependent-Care and Nursing, 16*(1), 41–48.

Schön, D. (1987). *Educating the reflective practitioner: Toward a new design for teaching and learning in the professions.* Jossey-Bass.

Schön, D. (1991). *The reflective practitioner: How professionals think in action.* Ashgate.

Schön, D. (2009). *The reflective practitioner: How professionals think in action.* Ashgate.

Seedhouse, D., & Peuthrer, V. (2020). *Using personal judgement in nursing and healthcare* (1st ed.). Sage.

Sharkiya, S. H. (2023). Quality communication can improve patient-centred health outcomes among older patients: A rapid review. *BMC Health Services Research, 23,* 886.

Sherwood, G. (2024). Reflective practice and knowledge development: Transforming research for a practice-based discipline. *International Journal of Nursing Sciences, 11*(4), 399–404.

Smith, B., & Field, L. (2020). *Nursing care: An essential guide for nurses and healthcare workers in primary and secondary care* (3rd ed.). Routledge.

Smith, A., & Jack, K. (2005). Reflective practice: A meaningful task for students. *Nursing Standard, 19*(26), 33–37.

Standing, M. (2023). *Clinical judgement and decision-making for nursing students* (5th ed.). SAGE.

Stein, J. P., Koban, K., Joos, S., & Ohler, P. (2020). Worth the effort? Comparing different YouTube vlog production styles in terms of viewers' identification, parasocial response, immersion, and enjoyment. *Psychology of Aesthetics, Creativity, and the Arts.* Advance online publication. https://psycnet.apa.org/record/2020-90013-001

Stephenson, S., & Holm, D. (1994). Reflection: A student's perspective. In A. Palmer, S. Burns, & C. Bulman (Eds.), *Reflective practice in nursing: The growth of the professional practitioner* (p. 137). Blackwell Science.

Stevens, D. D., & Cooper, J. E. (2009). *Reflection and learning from experience in journal keeping: How to use reflective writing for learning, teaching, professional insight and positive change.* Stylus.

Stuart, P. (2022). How do hospital nurses experience end-of-life care provision? A creative phenomenological approach. *British Journal of Nursing, 31*(19), 997–1002.

Sundgren, M. K., Millear, P. M., Dawber, C., & Medoro, L. (2021). Reflective practice groups and nurse professional quality of life. *Australian Journal of Advanced Nursing, 38*(4), 49–67.

Taylor, B. (2010). *Reflective practice for healthcare professionals* (3rd ed.). Open University Press.

Taylor, J. A., Sims, J., & Hill, H. (2015). Reflective practice and its relationship to mindfulness, situation/movement awareness and person-centredness during mobility care in nursing homes: A discussion paper. *Reflective Practice, 16*(4), 449–458.

Thobaben, M. (2007). Horizontal workplace violence. *Home Care Management and Practice, 20,* 82–83.

Thompson, S., & Thompson, N. (2023). *The critically reflective practitioner* (3rd ed.). Bloomsbury.

Trueland, J. (2022). Supervision and keeping the relationship positive. *Nursing Standard, 37*(6), 24–26.

Turkel, M. C., Watson, J., & Giovannoni, J. (2018). Caring science or science of caring. *Nursing Science Quarterly, 31*(1), 66–67.

United Kingdom Central Council (UKCC) for Nursing, Midwifery and Health Visiting. (1994). *The future of professional practice: The council's standard for education and practice following registration.* UKCC.

van Ooijen, E. (2013). *Clinical supervision made easy* (2nd ed.). PCCS Books.

Voldbjerg, S. L., Wiechula, R., Elgaard Sørensen, E., & Grønkjær, M. (2021). Newly graduated nurses' socialisation resulting in limiting inquiry and one-sided use of knowledge sources—An ethnographic study. *Journal of Clinical Nursing, 30*(5–6), 701–711. https://doi.org/10.1111/jocn.15592

Watson, J. (1988). *Nursing: Human science and human care: A theory of nursing.* National League for Nursing.

Watson, J. (2008). *Nursing: The philosophy and science of caring* (Rev. ed.). University Press of Colorado.

Watson, N. A. (2024). *Effective communication for nursing practice.* Learning Matters.

West, L. (2001). *Doctors on the edge: General practitioners' health and learning in the inner city.* Free Associates Books.

Williamson, G. R., Kane, A., Plowright, H., Bunce, J., Clarke, D., & Jamison, C. (2020). Thinking like a nurse': Changing the culture of nursing students' clinical learning: Implementing collaborative learning in practice. *Nurse Education in Practice, 43.* Article 102706.

Willis, P. (2015). Raising the bar. Shape of caring: A review of the future education and training of registered nurses and care assistants. *HEE in association with the NMC.* https://www.hee.nhs.uk/sites/default/files/documents/2348-Shape-of-caring-review-FINAL.pdf

Winnicott, D. W. (1965). *The maturational processes and the facilitating environment: Studies in the theory of emotional development.* Karnac and the Institute of Psycho-Analysis.

Xu, Y., & Davidhizar, R. (2005). Intercultural communication in nursing education: When Asian students and American faculty converge. *Journal of Nursing Education, 44*(5), 209–215.

Zander, P. E. (2007). Ways of knowing in nursing: The historical evolution of a concept. *Journal of Theory Construction & Testing, 11*(1), 7–11.

Zonneveld, D., Conroy, T., & Lines, L. (2024). Clinical supervision experience of nurses in or transitioning to advanced practice: A systematic review. *Journal of Advanced Nursing, 80*(9), 3547–3564.

# Index